Advanced Disaster Medical Response Manual for Providers
Second Edition

Susan Miller Briggs MD, MPH, FACS
Editor

DEDICATION

In memory of the victims of disasters throughout the world, including the tragic Boston Marathon terrorist attack in 2013.

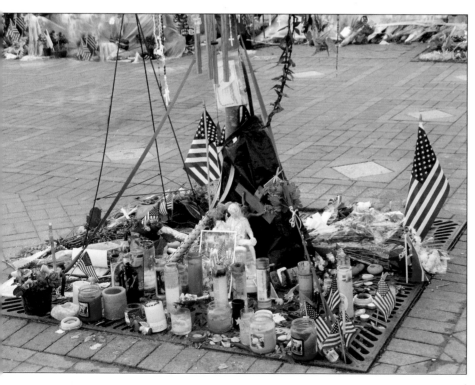

Memorial to Victims of Boston Marathon Bombing

PUBLISHED BY:

Ciné-Med Publishing, Inc.
127 Main Street North
Woodbury, CT 06798
(203) 263-0006
Copyright© 2014

ISBN: 978-1-941805-01-5

Notice: Our knowledge in clinical sciences is constantly changing. As new information becomes available, changes in treatment and in the use of drugs or medical devices become necessary. The authors and the publisher of this volume have taken care to make certain that the doses of drugs, uses of medical devices, and schedules of treatment are correct and compatible with the standards generally accepted at the time of publication.

Printed in Canada

EDITOR

SUSAN MILLER BRIGGS, MD, MPH, FACS
Associate Professor of Surgery, Harvard Medical School

Director, International Trauma and Disaster Institute,
Department of Surgery, Massachusetts General Hospital
Boston, Massachusetts

Affiliate Faculty, Department of Global Health and Social Medicine,
Program in Global Surgery and Social Change, Harvard Medical School
Boston, Massachusetts

Editor, American Journal of Disaster Medicine

Past-President, Panamerican Trauma Society

The authors would like to thank the Flatley Foundation for their support of this project and their continuing commitment to the care of victims of disasters throughout the world.

ACKNOWLEDGMENTS

The author gratefully acknowledges the contributions of the Assistant Editors. Their professional expertise and disaster experience contributed significantly to making the Second Edition of the Advanced Disaster Medical Response Manual a valuable educational resource for disaster providers.

ASSISTANT EDITORS

Roy Alson MD

Edward George MD

David Lawlor MD

Conrad Salinas MD

Joseph Scott MD

CONSULTANTS

The author would also like to acknowledge the following consultants who provided invaluable support for the manual.

Jessica Briggs, *Graphic Design Consultant*

Michael Cronin, *Technical Consultant*

Jan van Steenwijk, *Photography Consultant*

CONTRIBUTING AUTHORS

Roy L. Alson, MD, PhD, FACEP
Associate Professor, Department of Emergency Medicine,
Wake Forest University School of Medicine, Winston-Salem, NC
Medical Director, State Medical Response System, NC Office of EMS,
Raleigh, North Carolina

William Beninati, MD, FCCP
Colonel, US Air Force (Retired)
Adjunct Assistant Professor of Medicine,
University of Utah School of Medicine
Assistant Medical Director for Critical Care, Intermountain Life Flight,
LSD Hospital, Salt Lake City, Utah

Jeffrey N. Bernstein, MD
Voluntary Associate Professor of Pediatrics and Medicine,
University of Miami Miller School of Medicine
Medical Director, Florida Poison Information Center/Miami
Attending Physician, Emergency Care Center
Jackson Memorial Hospital, Miami, Florida

Arthur M. Bohanan, BS, CLPE
Forensic Examiner, Sevierville Police Department
President, Tennessee Cadaver Research Institute
Disaster Mortuary Operational Response Team (DMORT) -
Weapons of Mass Destruction Team (WMD) - (Retired)
New Market, Tennessee

Christopher T.Born, MD, FAAOS, FACS
Intrepid Heroes Professor of Orthopaedic Surgery
Chief, Orthopaedic Trauma
Brown University, Providence, Rhode Island

Eileen M. Bulger, MD, FACS
Professor of Surgery, University of Washington,
Chief of Trauma, Harborview Medical Center,
Seattle, Washington

Christine Curci, PhD, MSW, LCSW
Consultant, Mental Health and Conflict Mitigation,
Cumberland, Maine

Arup De, MD
Assistant Professor of Anesthesiology, Chief of Clinical Anesthesia,
South Clinical Campus, Albany Medical Center, Albany, New York

Edward M. Eitzen, MD, MPH
Colonel, US Army (Retired)
Senior Partner, Biodefense and Public Health Programs,
Martin- Blanck and Associates
Alexandria, Virginia

Peter J. Fagenholz, MD
Instructor in Surgery, Harvard Medical School
Assistant in Surgery, Department of Trauma, Emergency Surgery and
Surgical Critical Care, Massachusetts General Hospital
Affiliate Faculty, Department of Global Health and Social Medicine,
Harvard Medical School, Boston, Massachusetts

CONTRIBUTING AUTHORS (cont.)

Brian W. Flynn, Ed.D
Associate Director, Center for Studies of Traumatic Stress
Adjunct Professor of Psychiatry, Department of Psychiatry
Uniformed Services University of the Health Sciences, (USUHS),
Bethesda, Maryland

Anthony J. Forgione, LPN, CST
Surgical Technology Instructor, Quincy College, Quincy, Massachusetts
Surgical Technologist/ LPN, Massachusetts General Hospital
President, Boston Chapter, National Association of Orthopedic Nurses
Boston, Massachusetts

Edward E. George, MD, PhD
Commander, US Navy Reserve
Assistant Professor of Anesthesia, Harvard Medical School
Medical Director, Post-Anesthesia Care Units,
Department of Anesthesia and Critical Care,
Massachusetts General Hospital, Boston, Massachusetts

Annekathryn Goodman, MD, FACS, FACOG
Associate Professor of Obstetrics, Gynecology and Reproductive Biology,
Harvard Medical School
Department of Obstetrics and Gynecology,
Massachusetts General Hospital
Affiliate Faculty, Department of Global Health and Social Medicine.
Harvard Medical School, Boston, Massachusetts

N. Stuart Harris, MD, MFA
Assistant Professor of Surgery (Emergency Medicine),
Harvard Medical School
Chief, Division of Wilderness Medicine
Fellowship Director, MGH Wilderness Medicine Fellowship
Department of Emergency Medicine,
Massachusetts General Hospital, Boston, Massachusetts

Graham Ingalsbe, MD
University of Miami Miller School of Medicine, Miami, Florida

Mark E. Keim, MD
Associate Director for Science
Office for Environmental Health Emergencies
Centers for Disease Control and Prevention, Atlanta, Georgia

David F. Lawlor, MD, FACS
Instructor, Harvard Medical School
Department of Surgery, Division of Pediatric Surgery,
Massachusetts General Hospital
Affiliate Faculty, Department of Global Health and Social Medicine,
Harvard Medical School
Consulting Medical Staff, Shriners Hospital for Children
Boston, Massachusetts

Shannon F. Manzi, PharmD
Adjunct Assistant Professor, College of Pharmacy,
Massachusetts College of Pharmacy and Allied Health Services
Team Leader, Emergency Services, Department of Pharmacy,
Boston Children's Hospital, Boston, Massachusetts

Larry W. Masterman, MICP, CEM
Emergency Operations Manager,
Trinity County Office of Emergency Services
Managing Partner, Preparedness Consulting & Training, International
Weaverville, California

Mark P. McAndrew MD, FACS, FAAOS
Professor of Surgery, Southern Illinois University School of Medicine
Orthopaedics and Rehabilitation, Memorial Medical Center
Springfield, Illinois

Joseph A. Moretti, MD, FACS
Clinical Instructor, Otology and Laryngology, Harvard Medical School
(Retired), Surgeon Emeritus, Massachusetts Eye and Ear Infirmary
Boston, Massachusetts

Michael G. Morley, MD, MHCM
Assistant Clinical Professor of Ophthalmology, Harvard Medical School
Assistant Surgeon, Massachusetts Eye and Ear Institute
Clinical Associate, Massachusetts General Hospital
Boston, Massachusetts

Vicki E. Noble, MD, FACEP
Associate Professor of Surgery (Emergency Medicine),
Harvard Medical School
Director, Emergency Ultrasound Division, Massachusetts General Hospital
Boston, Massachusetts

Cory D. Oaks, EMT-Paramedic
Adjunct Faculty, Utah Fire and Rescue Academy
Fire Captain, Provo City Fire and Rescue, Utah
Flight Paramedic, Intermountain Life Flight, Salt Lake City, Utah

Daphne Morrison Ponce, MD
LT, US Navy Reserve
Harvard Associated Emergency Medicine Residency
Massachusetts General Hospital, Boston, Massachusetts

Eric M. Rudnick, MD, FACEP, FAAEM
Medical Director, Northern California Emergency Medical Services, Inc.
Medical Director, Santa Clara County Emergency Medical Services
Agency, Division of Public Health, Santa Clara, California

Conrad Salinas, MD
Clinical Assistant Professor of Emergency Medicine
College of Osteopathic Medicine of the Pacific
Department of Emergency Medicine, Loma Linda VA
Loma Linda, California

Christopher Sanford, MD, MPH, DTM&H
Associate Professor, Department of Family Medicine
Associate Professor, Department of Global Health
Director, Travel Clinic, UW Neighborhood Northgate Clinic
University of Washington School of Medicine, Seattle, Washington

Felipe Santos, MD
Instructor, Otology and Laryngology, Harvard Medical School
Assistant in Otolaryngology, Massachusetts Eye and Ear Infirmary
Clinical Associate, Otolaryngology, Massachusetts General Hospital
Boston, Massachusetts

CONTRIBUTING AUTHORS (cont.)

Joseph A. Scott, MD, FACEP, FAAEM
Chair, Department of Emergency Medicine, West Kendall Baptist Hospital
Clinical Assistant Professor, Florida International University
Wertheim College of Medicine, Miami, Florida

David V. Shatz, MD, FACS
Professor of Surgery, University of California, Davis School of Medicine,
Department of Surgery, University of California Davis Medical Center,
Sacramento, California

Robert L. Sheridan, MD, FACS
Colonel, US Army Reserve
Associate Professor of Surgery, Harvard Medical School
Director, Acute Burn Service, Shriners Hospital Children
Affiliate Faculty, Department of Global Health and Social Medicine,
Harvard Medical School, Boston, Massachusetts

Bradford J. Shingleton, MD
Associate Clinical Professor of Ophthalmology, Harvard Medical School
Clinical Instructor, Tufts University School of Medicine
Surgeon, Boston and Cape Cod Eye Surgery and Laser Centers
Clinical Associate, Massachusetts General Hospital, Boston, Massachusetts

N. Steve Tinder, BS
Deputy Commander Disaster Mortuary Operational Response Team
(DMORT) - Weapons of Mass Destruction Team (WMD)
Knoxville, Tennessee

Bruce K. Waite, DO, FACOOG
Department of Obstetrics and Gynecology,
Redington-Fairview General Hospital, Skowhegan, Maine

Frank G. Walter, MD, FACEP, FACMT, FAACT
Professor of Emergency Medicine & Director of Clinical Toxicology,
Department of Emergency Medicine
Editor, Advanced Hazmat Life Support (AHLS)
Arizona Emergency Medical Research Center
The University of Arizona College of Medicine, Tucson, Arizona

Debra L. Weiner, MD, PhD, FAAP
Assistant Professor of Pediatrics, Harvard Medical School
Attending Physician, Division of Emergency Medicine,
Boston Children's Hospital, Boston, Massachusetts

Richard S. Weisman Pharm.D
Professor of Pediatrics, Associate Dean for Admissions
University of Miami Miller School of Medicine
Director, Florida Poison Information Center, University of Miami/Jackson
Memorial Medical Center, Miami, Florida

Kevin S. Yeskey, MD, FACEP
Senior Advisor for Emergency Public Health MDB, Inc.
Former Deputy Assistant Secretary for Preparedness and Response
Former Director, Office of Preparedness and Emergency Operations
Department of Health and Human Services, Washington, DC

TABLE OF CONTENTS

Mass Casualty Incident Management

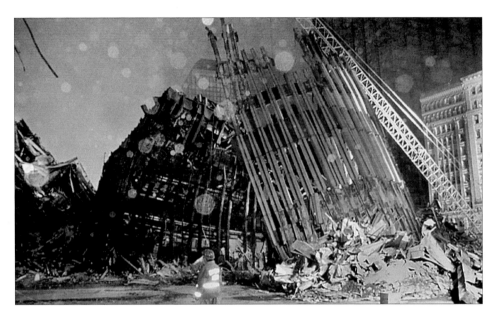

Fig. 1.1 World Trade Center terrorist attack, New York (2001)

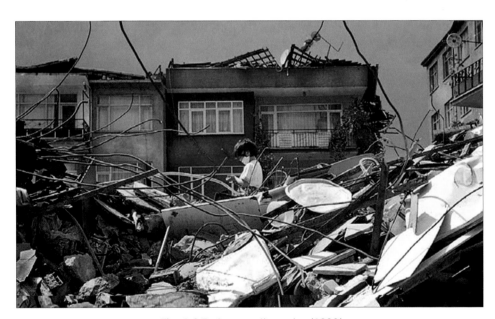

Fig. 1.2 Turkey earthquake (1999)

Introduction

Contemporary disasters follow no rules. No one can predict the time, location, or complexity of the next disaster. The management of the medical and public health effects of contemporary disasters, whether natural or man-made, is one of the most significant challenges facing medical providers today. Disaster medical care is **NOT** the same as conventional medical care. Disaster medical care requires a fundamental change in the care of disaster victims in order to achieve the objective of providing the "greatest good for the greatest number of victims." **DEMAND FOR RESOURCES ALWAYS EXCEEDS THE SUPPLY OF RESOURCES IN A MASS CASUALTY INCIDENT (MCI).**

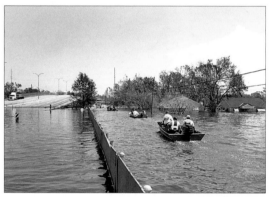

Fig. 1.3 Hurricane Katrina, New Orleans (2005)

Mass casualty incidents are events causing numbers of casualties large enough to disrupt the healthcare services of the affected community. The demands of disaster medical relief have changed over the past decade, both in the scope of medical care, the spectrum of threats, and the field of operations. Increasingly, medical providers are being asked to respond to complex disasters, with the spectrum of threats ranging from natural disasters to complex man-made disasters such as war and terrorism. Many of today's disasters occur or result in "austere" environments. Access, transport, resources, or other aspects of the physical, social, or economic environments may impose severe constraints on the adequacy of immediate care to the population in need.

Epidemiology of Disasters

Natural disasters may be classified as sudden-impact (acute) disasters or chronic-onset (slow) disasters. Sudden-impact natural disasters generally cause significant morbidity and mortality immediately as a direct result of the primary event (e.g., traumatic injuries, crush injuries, drowning). Chronic-onset disasters cause mortality and morbidity through prolonged secondary effects (e.g.,infectious disease outbreaks, dehydration, malnutrition).

2

Man-made disasters may be unintentional or intentional (terrorism) and range from technological disasters to MCI involving weapons of mass destruction (radioactive, biological, and chemical agents).

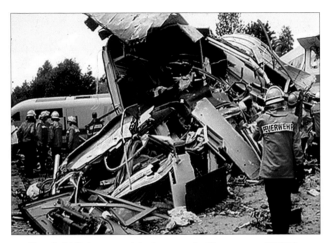

Fig. 1.4 High-speed train wreck, Germany (1998)

Disasters involving weapons of mass destruction (WMD) are a significant challenge for all disaster responders for the following reasons:

- WMD have the potential to produce casualties in numbers large enough to overwhelm healthcare systems.

- WMD may produce large numbers of **"expectant" victims** (individuals not expected to survive due to severity of injuries or underlying diseases and/or limited resources).

- WMD may produce a **contaminated environment**. Responders must be able to perform triage, initial stabilization, and possibly definitive care outside traditional healthcare facilities.

- WMD often produce significant numbers of **psychogenic casualties**.

The spectrum of agents used by terrorists is limitless and includes conventional weapons, explosives, and biological, chemical, and radioactive agents. 70% of terrorist attacks involve the use of explosive weapons and are a significant challenge for medical providers due to the complexity of injuries (primary, secondary, tertiary, and quaternary blast injuries). Terrorists do not have to kill people to achieve their goals. They just have to create a climate of fear and panic to overwhelm the healthcare system (examples: sarin/anthrax attacks).

Principles of Disaster Response

Lessons from previous disasters are important in distinguishing **"myths"** (misconceptions) from **"facts"** (evidence-based data).

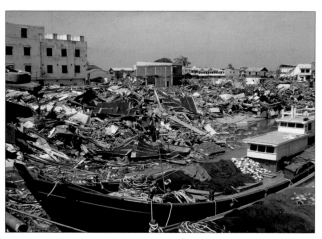

Fig. 1.5 Tsunami, Indonesia (2004)

Disaster Myth #1: Disaster responders can utilize traditional command structures when participating in disaster response.

- **Lesson Learned:** The Incident Command System (ICS) is the accepted standard for all disaster response. **Functional requirements, not titles, determine the organizational structure of the ICS.**

Disaster Myth #2: All disasters are different and require unique disaster plans to meet the medical and public health challenges of the specific disaster.

- **Lesson Learned:** Disaster response includes basic elements that are similar In all disasters.

MEDICAL CONCERNS:

- Search and rescue
- Triage
- Definitive care
- Evacuation

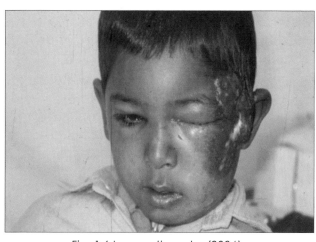

Fig. 1.6 Iran earthquake (2004)

4

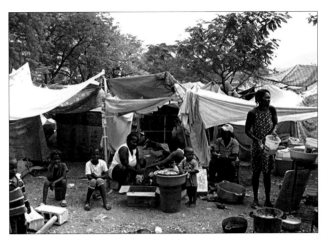

Fig. 1.7 Haiti earthquake (2010)

The difference in disasters is the degree of disruption of public health and medical services and the degree to which outside assistance (regional, national, or international) is required to respond to the needs of disaster victims. Rapid assessment by experienced disaster responders will determine which of these elements are needed in the acute phase of the disaster to augment local capacities. Factors determining whether an MCI overwhelms the medical and/or public health infrastructure of the community include the number, severity, and diversity of injuries. **Disaster management teams must be based on "functional" capacities, not titles.**

Disaster Myth #3: *Effective "surge capacity" is based on well-intentioned and readily available volunteers.*

- **Lesson Learned:** Responders must understand the basic principles of disaster response (ICS, disaster triage, gross decontamination) to be effective members of the disaster team. Responders must be willing to care for non-disaster-related diseases/emergencies as well as disaster–related injuries. **TRAINING IS AN ESSENTIAL PART OF DISASTER PREPAREDNESS.**

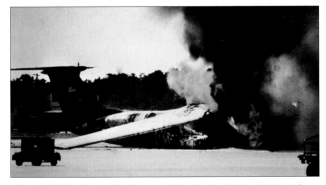

Fig. 1.8 Disaster training must include the response to hazardous-material incidents.

Disaster Myth #4: Disaster medical care is the same as conventional medical care.

- **Lesson Learned:** Disaster medical care requires a <u>fundamental</u> change in the approach to the care of victims **("crisis management care")**. The objective of disaster medical care is the greatest good for the greatest number of victims. This is in contrast to the objective of conventional medical care, which is the greatest good for the individual patient.

Disaster Myth #5: Politics do not dictate disaster response.

- **Lesson Learned:** Politics, more than lack of personnel, supplies, and equipment, limits the effectiveness of disaster preparedness and response to today's complex disasters.

Phases of Disaster Management

It is important to apply the principles of MCI management to all four phases of disaster management.

Phase 1: <u>Preparedness:</u> planning/training
Phase 2: <u>Mitigation:</u> hazard vulnerability
Phase 3: <u>Response:</u> emergency phase
Phase 4: <u>Recovery:</u> restoration

Disaster Drills

Disaster preparedness activities consist of making a community aware of possible disaster situations, training personnel, purchasing equipment to support response activities, marshaling resources, engaging in inter-agency planning, and conducting the full spectrum of community preparedness exercises. **Disaster preparedness must include practical drills to ascertain the true magnitude of system problems, not just tabletop exercises.** Mass-casualty drills must include three phases:

- <u>Preparation Phase</u>
- <u>Exercise Management Phase</u>
- <u>Patient Treatment Phase</u>

The **preparation phase** must include clear definition of functional areas of responsibility that can be evaluated objectively, not subjectively, during the disaster drill.

The **exercise management phase** includes objective evaluation of all key functional roles in the ICS.

The **patient treatment phase** includes objective evaluation of well-defined functional capacities such as:

- Triage
- Initial resuscitation
- Definitive care
- Evacuation
- Care of dead victims

Summary

A consistent approach to disasters, based on an understanding of their common features and the response expertise they require, is becoming the accepted practice throughout the world. This strategy, called the Mass Casualty Incident Response, has the primary objective of reducing the mortality and morbidity caused by the disaster. All medical personnel need to incorporate the key principles of the MCI response in their training, given the complexity of today's disasters.

The goal of disaster medical response is to reduce the critical mortality associated with a disaster. **Critical mortality rate is defined as the percentage of critically injured survivors who subsequently die.** Numerous factors influence the critical mortality rate, including:

- Triage accuracy, particularly the incidence of over-triage of victims
- Rapid movement of patients to definitive care
- Implementation of damage control procedures
- Coordinated regional disaster preparedness

KEY POINTS

 The demand for resources always exceeds the supply of resources in a mass casualty incident.

 Disaster medical care is NOT the same as conventional medical care.

 Disaster preparedness must include practical drills, not just tabletop exercises.

 Disaster management teams are based on functional capacities, not titles.

Incident Command System

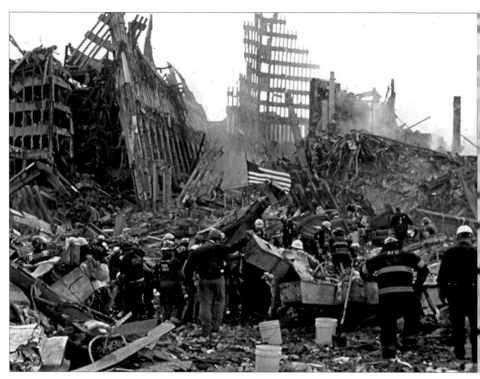

Fig. 2.1 World Trade Center terrorist attack, New York (2001)

CASE SCENARIO

On September 11, 2001, hijackers intentionally crashed two fully fueled planes into the Twin Towers of the World Trade Center in New York City, the result of a coordinated terrorist attack on the United States. More than 2,500 people died and over 3,000 individuals were injured. Both of the Twin Towers collapsed after the attack, significantly adding to the mortality and morbidity of the disaster. An effective Incident Command System (ICS) helped to coordinate federal, state, and local assets responding to the disaster.

Introduction

Disasters bring together organizations from different jurisdictions and disciplines. It is critical that an integrated command and control system be established so that all responders can function in a coordinated, safe, and effective manner. The methodology used to achieve this in North America and other parts of the world is the Incident Command System/Incident Management System. **The ICS is widely recognized as an effective method of managing all organizations, including hospitals, that respond to a disaster.**

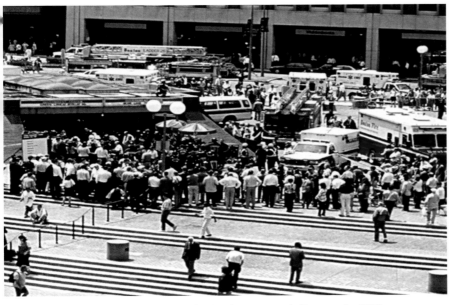

Fig. 2.2 Efficient, coordinated response is the goal of ICS.

The current model of ICS grew out of the Firescope program developed in the United States in the 1970s to deal with wildfires in California that involved multiple agencies at the federal, state, and local levels. Review of previous events showed that lack of common operating procedures resulted in poorly coordinated disaster operations with increased injuries and property losses. The goal of ICS is to simplify communications and establish clear lines of authority and responsibility. ICS has been adopted as the standard command system for all mass casualty incidents in North America.

The Incident Command System offers the following advantages:

- **Flexible:** It can be used for any type of event (fires, earthquakes, planned events, etc).
- **Scalable:** It can be used for any-size event.

- **Adaptable:** As conditions change during an event, ICS can be configured to meet those changes.
- **Sustainable:** ICS can be used for extended periods as transfer of command is an integral component.

ICS Structure

The ICS is a modular/adaptable system for all incidents and facilities. **Functional requirements, not titles, determine the ICS hierarchy.** The organizational structure of the ICS is built around five major management activities (Incident Command, Operations, Planning, Logistics, and Finance/Administration).

SUBJECT MATTER EXPERTS

The Incident Commander may appoint various subject-matter experts (SME) to assist with the operation.

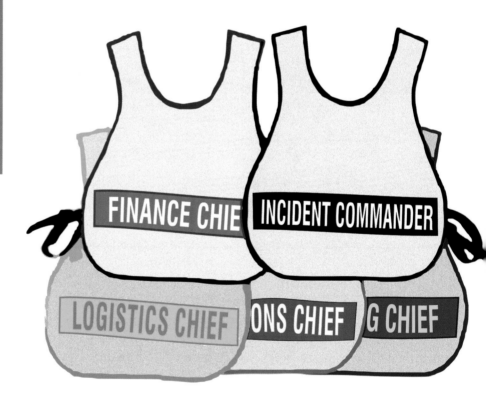

Fig. 2.3 ICS

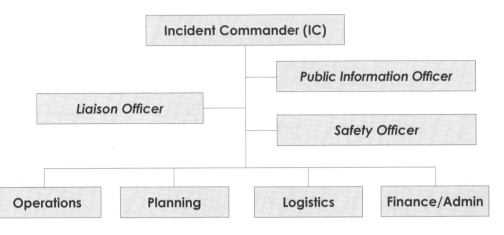

INCIDENT COMMANDER	• Sets objectives and priorities
	• Maintains overall responsibility for the incident
	• May appoint a Deputy Commander
	• The IC Is assisted by the following:
	   ◦ **Liaison Officer**—coordinates efforts with other agencies and jurisdictions
	   ◦ **Public Information Officer**—deals with the press and the public, ensuring that effective risk-management messages are transmitted
	   ◦ **Safety Officer**—ensures the safety of responders

OPERATIONS	• Conducts operations to carry out Incident Action Plan(s) • Directs all disaster resources, including medical personnel
PLANNING	• Develops Incident Action Plans • Collects/evaluates information • Maintains resource status
LOGISTICS	• Provides resources and support to meet incident needs, including responder needs
FINANCE AND ADMINISTRATION	• Monitors costs • Executes contracts • Provides legal advice • Maintains records of personnel

Some characteristics of the ICS that enable it to be used effectively in a disaster include the following:

- The ICS uses a common terminology for positions, functions, and resources, thereby eliminating confusion. This enhances communication across jurisdictions and disciplines.

- There is unity of command, meaning that each person reports to <u>only one</u> person, and there is a single commander for the incident.

- The command structure for the event is delineated so that authority and responsibilities are understood, as is the chain of command. Furthermore, there are defined procedures to transfer command.

- The use of the ICS allows for establishing a Unified Command when multiple agencies or jurisdictions are involved.

- The modular nature of the system allows it to expand or contract to deal with all sizes of incidents and hazards.

- The use of the ICS allows tracking of assets and personnel at the event, reducing risks to responders and allowing for effective utilization of available resources.

One of the central tenets of the ICS is **"management by objectives"**. The system attempts to bring "best practices" to the management of an incident. Individuals or units are assigned specific tasks that are defined and have measurable outcomes. Furthermore, each assignment also allocates the resources that are available to allow completion of the task. All of these are spelled out in the Incident Action Plan (IAP), which allows for effective communication of the incident objectives and assignments to all participants.

Span of control is another important concept within the ICS. **No one individual should supervise more than 7 subordinates so that effective lines of communication can be maintained.**

Integration into Unified Command

Each organization brings its own ICS to the disaster. As the incident enlarges, Unified Command is formed, allowing all organizations to work together under a single command structure. Examples of unified command structure include:

- Establishing a single command center with police, emergency medical services, and fire at a major hazardous-materials incident.

- Coordination of the public information officers into a Joint Information Center (JIC), so that the press and public receive consistent and timely information.

SPAN OF CONTROL

Each person within the command structure should supervise between three and seven (3-7) persons.

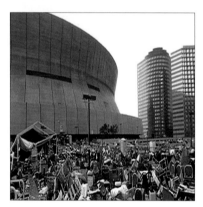

Fig. 2.4 Hurricane Katrina, New Orleans (2005) highlighted the need for an effective ICS to coordinate multiple responding agencies.

Important Principles

- The ICS needs to be started early, before an incident gets out of control. Some experts say that for every five minutes an incident continues before the ICS is implemented, it takes a half hour longer to bring the incident under control.

- Medical responders, often used to working independently, must adhere to the structure of an ICS in order to integrate successfully into the rescue effort.

- When there are multiple injuries or other medical concerns, it is imperative that EMS/Medical is part of Unified Command.

- Functional needs of the event determine positions within the command structure, not titles.

- For the operation to run effectively, appropriate information must be recorded and passed between commanders and others in the ICS at the change of shifts.

- **The structure of the ICS is the same regardless of the nature of the disaster.** The difference is in the particular experience of key personnel. In a biological incident, for example, key personnel would be experienced in infection control.

RISK ALERT!

Medical responders must adhere to the ICS structure to avoid many negative consequences, including:

- **Death of medical personnel due to lack of safety and training**
- **Lack of adequate medical supplies to provide care**
- **Staff working beyond their training or certification**

Summary

Today's disasters often require responses by multiple agencies from different jurisdictions. In order to effectively coordinate these resources and establish clear lines of authority, the ICS was established. The Hospital Incident Command System (HICS) is a specific adaptation of the ICS to hospitals and medical facilities. The structure of the ICS is the same regardless of the nature of the incident. The difference is in the particular experience of key personnel. The ICS can be expanded or contracted in a specific incident to meet changing needs of the disaster response.

KEY POINTS

The ICS is a modular/adaptable system for all incidents and facilities.

Functional requirements, not titles, determine the organizational hierarchy of the ICS structure.

The five critical areas involved in the ICS are Incident Command, Operations, Planning, Logistics, and Finance/Administration.

Search and Rescue

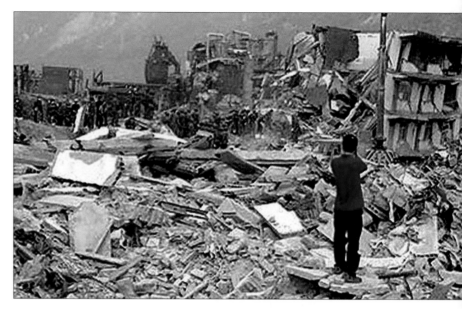

Fig. 3.1 Sichuan earthquake, China (2008)

CASE SCENARIO

On May 12, 2008, an 8.0 earthquake occurred in Sichuan Provinc China. More than 70,000 individuals died, over 370,000 victi were injured, and over 18,000 people are still missing. Casualt were initially treated at triage sites in the disaster region and th evacuated to hospitals throughout China. Numerous search a rescue teams were deployed to the disaster sites. Rescue effo were hampered by the austere geographic conditions, landslid flooding, and numerous aftershocks.

Introduction

The local population near any disaster site is the immediate search and rescue asset. Unfortunately, the local response is usually unsophisticated and haphazard, lacking the technical equipment and expertise to facilitate extrication of victims trapped in the rubble.

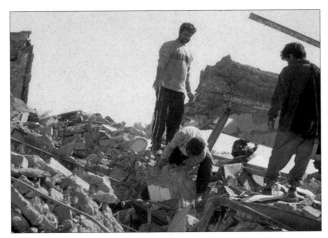

*Fig. 3.2 Immediate search and rescue efforts
by local population, Iran earthquake (2003)*

Many countries have developed specialized search and rescue teams such as the Urban Search and Rescue Teams (USAR) in the United States. USAR involves the location, rescue (extrication), and initial medical stabilization of victims trapped in "confined spaces". Search and rescue teams respond to a broad range of disasters, including earthquakes, mine collapses, bombings, and hurricanes such as Irene and Sandy.

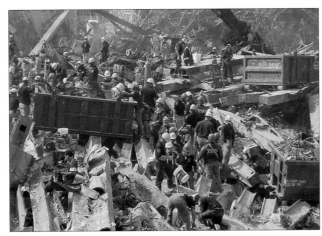

*Fig. 3.3 USAR teams, fire and police personnel
removing debris by hand and heavy machinery,
Ground Zero, New York (2001)*

Team Structure

Search and rescue teams are generally composed of specialists in the following areas:

- Technical search
- Disaster medicine
- Hazardous materials
- Communications and logistics
- Trained canines and their handlers

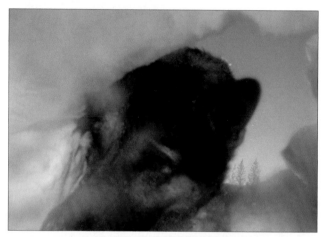

Fig. 3.4 Courtesy of FEMA

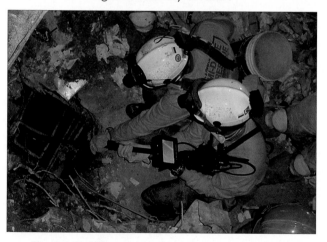

Fig. 3.5 Canine and technical search specialists attempting to locate victims

Team size varies depending on the country and sponsoring organizations (military or civilian). In the United States, there are currently 28 active USAR teams. Some or all of these teams can be activated simultaneously or staggered, depending on the magnitude of the event. Teams consist of over 200 personnel, with 30 to 75 mobilized for any given deployment, depending on the magnitude of the disaster and local capacities for search and rescue.

All team members spend an extensive amount of time in specialized training, not only in their own areas of expertise, but also **cross-training in the other areas** that the team is able to provide. While some of the removal of collapsed buildings and access to entrapped victims can be accomplished with heavy equipment such as bulldozers and cranes, much of the access and extrication is performed by hand by rescue specialists, with several hours often spent on a single victim.

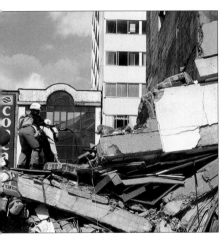 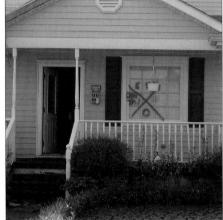

Figs. 3.6, 3.7 USAR teams

Team Activation

USAR team activities are highly coordinated in order to successfully extricate a live victim. The task of transporting 70 or more personnel and canines, as well as over 60,000 pounds of equipment, to locations throughout the world is a formidable one accomplished by logistics personnel. **Planning specialists update search locations and team movements throughout the deployment and decide which sections of the building or city should be searched next.**

Once an area has been chosen to focus efforts upon, search operations are begun to locate potential victims. Specially trained and nationally certified search dogs and their handlers, both in live-find and cadaver retrieval, are deployed. A potential "hit" by one dog is normally confirmed by another before additional resources are brought in.

17

Technical search equipment can be used to locate or confirm a victim buried behind or below concrete walls. Once located, rescue personnel move in with both a cadre of tools and their gloved hands. Before extrication proceeds too far, medical evaluation and treatment are begun. Victims are often immobile for several days and are subject to crush syndrome. Fully extricating a victim without proper medical intervention can lead to fatal results. Once mobilized and removed from the collapsed structure, victims are transported by pre-arranged rescue vehicles to mobile hospitals or hospitals that remain functional after the disaster event. USAR team members remain on-site unless the victim is a member of the team itself. The process is repeated for many days, with the hope of as many live-victim finds as possible.

At some point during the process, the likelihood of finding surviving victims diminishes. The ongoing significant risk to USAR personnel carrying out these operations in unstable structures converts the rescue operation to one of body recovery. Though always a difficult decision, teams have personally witnessed the concept of "closure" among family members when loved ones, though not among the survivors, are located and removed from the structure.

Summary

An important operational concept among all search and rescue teams is that their presence is one of support for local authorities, All decisions regarding operational management of the scene are the responsibility and privilege of the local agencies and authorities. No one knows the scene as well as those who live and work there, and their decisions are always to be respected.

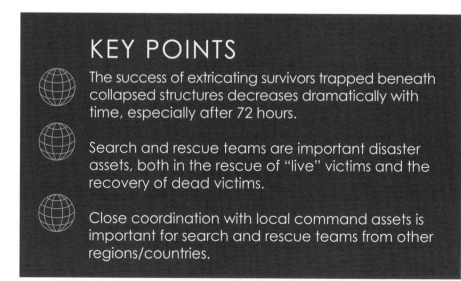

KEY POINTS

- The success of extricating survivors trapped beneath collapsed structures decreases dramatically with time, especially after 72 hours.

- Search and rescue teams are important disaster assets, both in the rescue of "live" victims and the recovery of dead victims.

- Close coordination with local command assets is important for search and rescue teams from other regions/countries.

Triage

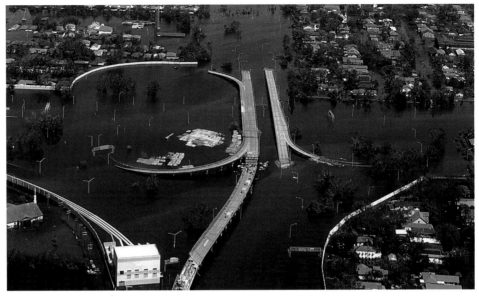

Fig. 4.1 Flooded City of New Orleans, Hurricane Katrina (2005)

CASE SCENARIO

Hurricane Katrina impacted much of the Gulf Coast of the United States, but the City of New Orleans, Louisiana, sustained some of the most devastating damage, both from the hurricane and multiple breaches to the levees. All hospitals in New Orleans were flooded or damaged and not available for medical care. Temporary triage stations were established throughout the city, including the airport, and staffed by mobile disaster teams, both civilian and military. Large numbers of casualties were ultimately evacuated due to the lack of functioning medical facilities in the city.

Introduction

Triage is the process of prioritizing casualties according to the level of care they require. It is the most important, and psychologically most difficult, mission of disaster medical response, both in the pre-hospital and hospital phases of the disaster. Disaster triage is significantly different from conventional civilian triage. **Disaster triage requires a fundamental change in the approach to the care of patients ("crisis management care").**

The objective of conventional civilian triage is to do the greatest good for the individual patient. Severity of injury/disease is the major determinant for medical care.

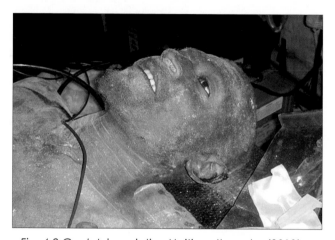

Fig. 4.2 Crush Injury victim, Haiti earthquake (2010)

The objective of disaster triage is to do the greatest good for the greatest number of patients. The determinants of triage in disasters are, however, based on three parameters:

• **Severity of injury**

• **Likelihood of survival**

• **Available resources (logistics, personnel, evacuation assets.)**

The major objective and challenge of triage is to rapidly identify the small minority of critically injured patients who require urgent life-saving interventions from the larger majority of non-critical casualties that characterize most disasters.

In a mass casualty event, the <u>critical</u> patients with the <u>greatest chance of survival</u> with the <u>least expenditure of time and resources</u> are prioritized to be treated first.

Triage is a dynamic decision-making process of matching victims' needs with available resources. Many mass casualty incidents will have <u>multiple</u> different levels of triage as patients move from the disaster scene to definitive medical care. **Disaster medical triage may be conducted at three different levels depending on the level of casualties (injuries) to capabilities (resources).**

Field Triage

Field triage, often the initial triage system utilized at the disaster scene in mass casualty incidents, is the rapid categorization of victims potentially needing immediate medical care "where they are laying" or at triage sites. **Victims are designated as "acute" or "non-acute." Simplified color coding may be used.**

Acute = RED

Non-acute = GREEN

One effective way to begin field triage with a large number of victims is to instruct individuals who can walk to get up and move to a designated location. This quickly separates the ambulatory (non-acute) from the non-ambulatory victims (acute) who cannot walk or talk. Once the victims are transported to casualty collection centers (fixed or mobile medical facilities), medical triage according to severity of injury may be performed.

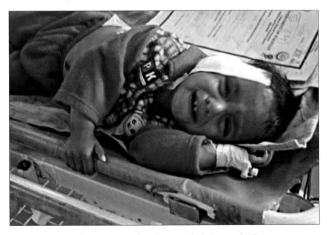

*Fig. 4.3 Pediatric crush injury victim,
Pakistan earthquake (2005)*

21

Medical Triage

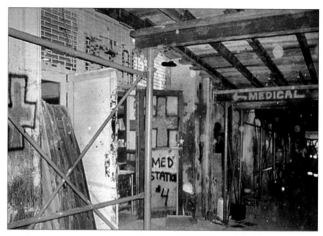

Fig. 4.4 Triage station, Ground Zero, New York (2001)

Medical triage is the rapid categorization of victims, at a casualty collection site or fixed or mobile medical facilities, by the most experienced medical personnel available to identify the level of medical care needed based on severity of injury. Triage personnel must have knowledge of the medical consequences of various injuries (e.g., burn, blast, or crush injuries or exposure to chemical, biological, or radioactive agents). Color coding may be used:

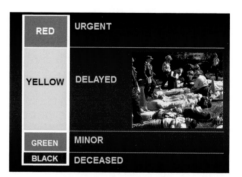

Fig. 4.5 Medical triage

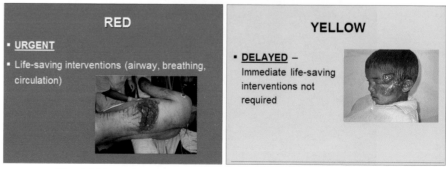

Fig. 4.6 Urgent care   *Fig. 4.7 Delayed care*

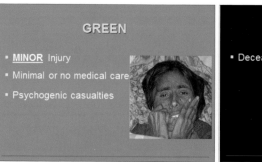

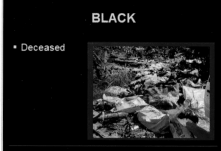

Fig. 4.8 Minimal care   Fig. 4.9 Dead victims

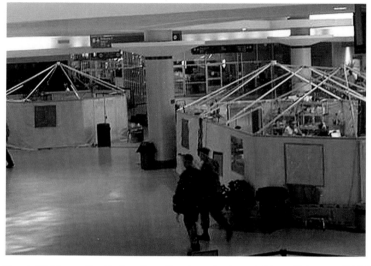

Fig. 4.10 Casualty Collection Center at airport, New Orleans (2005)

The **"expectant"** category of victims is unique to mass casualty incidents. Patients are classified as "expectant" victims if they are not expected to survive due to severity of injuries (massive crush injuries or severe total body surface area burns) or underlying diseases and/or limited resources. The "expectant" category of triage was first developed given the threat of weapons of mass destruction (biological, chemical, radioactive) during military conflicts.

Classification of the "expectant" category of disaster victims remains controversial. Historically, such victims were classified in the yellow or delayed category. Currently, most systems prefer to utilize a separate category as only palliative care will be administered to these patients. No universally accepted criteria exist for designation of victims to the "expectant" category. Many models have been proposed based on severity of injuries, age, underlying diseases, and hemodynamic stability of victims at time of rescue (cardiac arrest on scene, need for intubation, etc.).

Evacuation Triage

Evacuation triage assigns priorities to disaster victims for transfer to medical facilities. The goal is appropriate evacuation (by land or air) of victims according to severity of injury, likelihood of survival, and available resources.

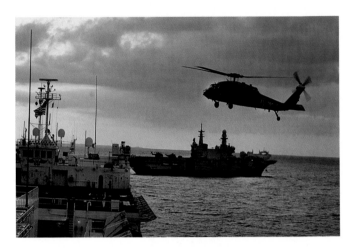

Fig. 4.11 Evacuation, Haiti earthquake (2010)

Triage Errors

Triage errors, in the form of over-triage and under-triage, are always present in the chaos of mass casualty events. **Over-triage** is the assignment of <u>non-critical survivors</u> with no life-threatening injuries to immediate <u>urgent</u> care. **Under-triage** is the assignment of <u>critically injured</u> casualties requiring immediate medical care to a <u>delayed</u> category.

The higher the incidence of over-triage of victims, the more the medical system is overwhelmed. Under-triage leads to delays in medical treatment with increased mortality and morbidity. In mass casualty incidents, especially explosions, triage errors more commonly involve over-triage than under-triage. Medical providers often over-triage children due to the emotional impact of injured children on medical personnel.

Triage Pitfalls

Triage pitfalls that lead to over-triage and under-triage include the following:

- No triage training prior to the disaster among medical personnel
- No standardized triage system among medical responders
- Selection of a triage officer lacking in rapid decision-making and leadership skills

24

- Failure to properly label patients by triage category, leading to triage redundancy, increased errors, and inefficiency
- Lack of personal protective equipment and communication tools to facilitate efficient triage in mass casualty incidents

Summary

Triage is never easy in disasters involving large numbers of casualties. Demand for resources always exceeds the supply of resources in a mass casualty incident. Triage is a dynamic process of matching patients' needs to available resources. **The goal of triage is to rapidly identify those victims with the greatest chance of survival given limited resources.**

KEY POINTS

The objective of disaster triage is to do the "greatest good for the greatest number of patients."

Triage in disasters is based on three parameters: severity of injuries, likelihood of survival and available resources.

Victims not expected to survive based on severity of injuries/underlying illnesses and/or available resources are classified as "expectant" victims in mass casualty incidents.

Definitive Medical Care

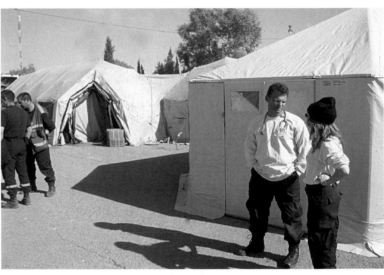

Fig.5.1 United States mobile hospital, Iran earthquake (2004)

CASE SCENARIO

A devastating 6.6 earthquake struck the city of Bam, Iran, in southeastern Iran on December 26, 2003. All medical facilities were destroyed, over 41,000 individuals killed, and tens of thousands injured. Thousands of victims were initially evacuated to Tehran, Iran, for definitive care. A request for international disaster relief was made by Iran. In addition to search and rescue teams and logistical supplies, 13 field hospitals, including a team from the United States, responded to the request to provide definitive medical care in Bam.

Introduction

Definitive medical care refers to care that will improve, rather than simply stabilize, a casualty's condition. Requirements for definitive medical care will vary widely depending on the magnitude and epidemiology of the disaster and the amount of destruction of the medical and public health infrastructure of the affected community/region. Both small-and large-scale disasters may require the mobilization of disaster medical teams to participate in the field medical response or supplement medical resources at fixed facilities in the disaster region. Alternatively, the evacuation of disaster victims to regional facilities outside the disaster region may be required to provide definitive care.

Crisis Management Care

The medical care that providers deliver in mass casualty incidents is significantly more austere than the care medical providers deliver on a day-to-day basis. **In mass casualty incidents, it is usually possible only to deliver "minimally acceptable care" or "crisis management care" in the initial phases of the disaster due to the large number of casualties.** Crisis management care focuses primarily on life-saving interventions in order to facilitate the "greatest good for the greatest number of victims." This is in contrast to the "maximally acceptable care" that is delivered in non-disaster situations.

Disaster Management Teams

The need for multi-disciplinary medical teams designed to augment existing medical resources at the time of a disaster is rapidly expanding due to the diversity and complexity of today's disaster threats. Current disaster preparedness and response emphasizes the need for an **All-Hazards** approach. Multi-disciplinary, mobile disaster teams that can provide a graded, flexible response to the need for definitive care in disasters are the key to an effective disaster response, especially if hospitals are destroyed or contaminated. The complexity of today's disasters demands civilian and military partnerships as key to effective disaster response.

Clinical competencies, not titles, determine the roles of medical providers in disaster response. Disaster management teams are designed and trained to provide specific **"functional"** areas of disaster care such as critical care, pediatrics, obstetrics, and acute and trauma surgery, especially when the casualty load is unknown.

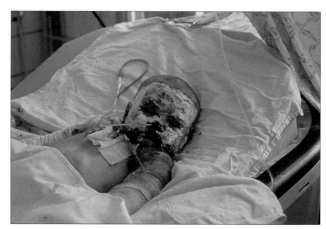

Fig. 5.2 Burn victim, Ufa, Russia train disaster (1989)

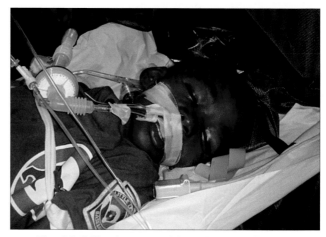

Fig. 5.3 Critical care, Haiti earthquake (2010)

Disaster management teams will vary depending on the etiology and complexity of the disaster. Most teams, however, include the following personnel:

- Team Commander
- Supervising Medical Officer
- Supervising Nurse
- Specialty Surgeons: trauma/orthopedics/plastics
- Emergency Medicine
- Anesthesia
- Critical Care
- Registered Nurses
- Medics
- Respiratory Therapists
- Logistics personnel, including pharmacy, biomedical, communication
- Security, Safety

Mobile Medical Facilities

Deployable, rapid-assembly medical facilities with the capacity for initial stabilization, operative interventions, and critical care are frequently used by both civilian and military medical teams and significantly increase the flexibility of the disaster response.

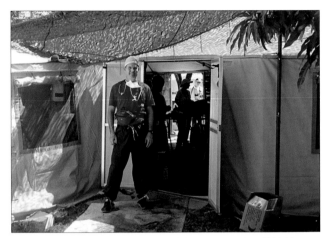

Fig 5.4 US field hospital, Haiti earthquake (2010)

In recent disasters such as the Indonesian tsunami and the Haiti earthquake, hospital ships have proven valuable definitive care assets.

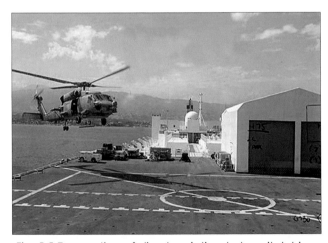

Fig. 5.5 Evacuation of disaster victims to hospital ship, USNS Comfort, Haiti (2010), Courtesy of US Navy.

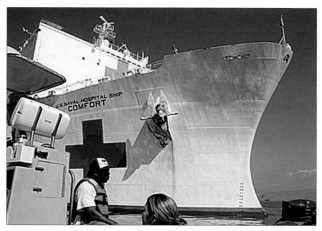

Fig 5.6 USNS Comfort, Haiti (2010), Courtesy of US Navy

Disaster Surgery

Damage control surgery is frequently employed in disaster settings and is an important component of crisis management care. In many disasters, local hospitals are destroyed, transportation to outside medical facilities may not be immediately feasible, or the environment may be contaminated, **Damage control surgery limits surgical interventions to control of hemorrhage and contamination.** This provides the opportunity to stabilize patients hemodynamically and correct hypothermia, acidosis and coagulopathy. Surgical patients can then undergo definitive repair of injuries at a later date. Damage control surgery was initially developed for abdominal trauma with uncontrolled hemorrhage, but has expanded to most other surgical specialties, such as orthopedic and vascular surgery.

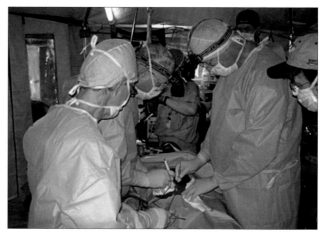

Fig. 5.7 Damage-control surgery,
Haiti earthquake (2010)

Mobile surgical facilities are important to provide a graded, flexible response to the need for surgical care. Surgical treatment is directed towards those individuals with the best chance of recovery with the least expenditure of resources, especially in austere environments. Spinal and regional anesthesia, as well as intravenous sedation, are important adjuvants to surgical therapy.

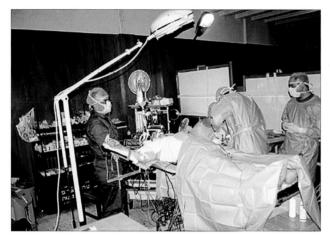

Fig 5.8 Definitive surgical care in schoolhouse,
Turkey earthquake (1999)

Sterilization of surgical instruments is a significant problem in mobile field hospitals. An accepted method of sterilizing instruments in austere environments is the use of Glutaraldehyde Solution 2%, a method utilized by many civilian and military field hospitals when conventional sterilization is not possible due to limited water and/or electricity.

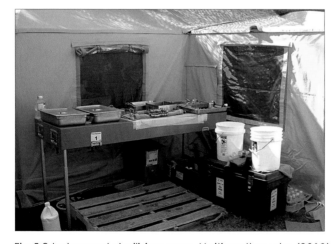

Fig 5.9 Instrument sterilizing area, Haiti earthquake (2010)

31

Summary

Disaster medical care requires specific knowledge of injury patterns commonly encountered in disasters, the professional skills to provide "crisis management care" in mass casualty incidents, and the ability to work as part of a multi-disciplinary, multi-organizational disaster response team.

KEY POINTS

 Maximally acceptable definitive care is rarely achieved in the initial phases of a mass casualty incident due to the large number of victims needing medical care.

 Damage control surgery is an important component of "crisis management care".

 Mobile multi-disciplinary medical teams with deployable field hospitals are valuable assets in disaster response, particularly in austere environments.

Evacuation

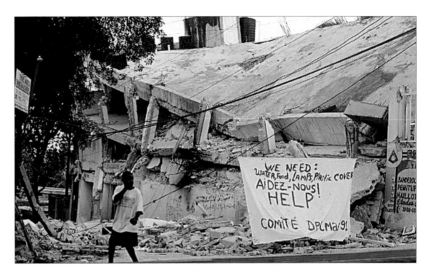

Fig. 6.1 Haiti earthquake (2010)

CASE SCENARIO

On January 12, 2010, a magnitude 7.0 earthquake occurred in Haiti, one of the poorest countries in the Western hemisphere. Port-au-Prince (PAP), the largest metropolis in Haiti, sustained devastating damage to the city, the airport, port facilities, and medical facilities, including all major hospitals. Greater than 200,000 people died, over 300,000 individuals were injured, and more than a million inhabitants were left homeless. Most roads were impassable due to the extensive earthquake damage. Evacuation of injured victims to medical facilities outside of the affected regions and international field hospitals in PAP was a major focus of disaster relief efforts.

Introduction

Evacuation can be useful in a disaster as a means of "decompressing" the disaster scene: removing the patients who are consuming the most resources. Evacuation of seriously injured casualties to off-site medical facilities not only improves their care, but also allows increased attention to remaining casualties at the disaster site.

There are significant patient stressors that accompany air evacuation, including changes in barometric pressure, decreased oxygen pressure, acceleration, vibration, turbulence, difficulty with environmental temperature control, reduced humidity, and noise. Careful pre-flight planning can minimize the effects of these stresses.

Indications for Evacuation

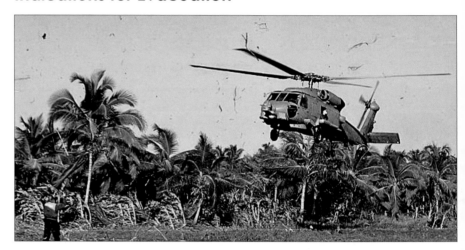

Fig. 6.2 Military helicopter assisting in rescue efforts in Haiti (2010), Courtesy of US Navy

There are several indications for evacuation in a disaster.

- To decompress the disaster area
    - o Critically ill patients consume disproportionate quantities of resources, including supplies, patient care space, and caregiver attention.
    - o Evacuating critical casualties allows the diversion of resources to a larger number of less critical casualties.
- To improve care for the most critical patients
    - o Minimize allocation of scarce resources to unstable patients by moving critical casualties to relatively resource-rich areas.
- To provide specialized care to specific casualties, such as those with burns and crush injuries

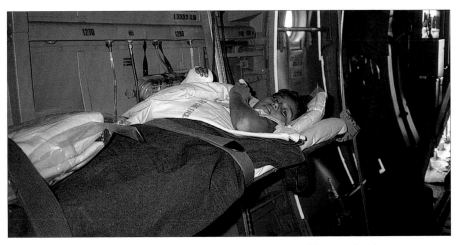

*Fig. 6.3 Interior of a military transport converted for medical use,
El Salvador earthquake (1987)*

Contraindications to Evacuation

There are several reasons to delay or defer evacuation of some casualties. These include:

- Contaminated casualties

  o Decontaminated victims can be marked by wristbands or other predetermined methods to ensure rescuer safety.

- Casualties with transmissible diseases
- Unstable casualties
- Lack of consent/diplomatic clearance

Modes of Evacuation

Ground

- Simple and generally available
- Inefficient – small numbers of casualties at once
- May remove critical resources from rescue efforts in the disaster area
- Buses may be used for mass transit of casualties who are triaged to a minimal care level.

Rotary-wing Aircraft and Small Fixed-wing Aircraft

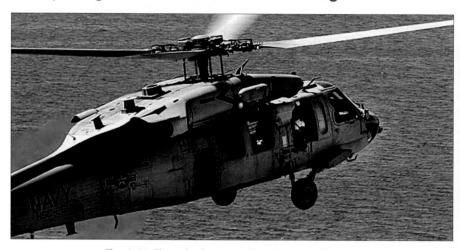

Fig. 6.4 Military helicopter, Courtesy of US Navy

- High cost and complexity
- Inefficient – small numbers of casualties at once
- Difficult to provide advanced care
- Aircraft may be better utilized in the disaster area for other purposes.

Large fixed-wing Aircraft

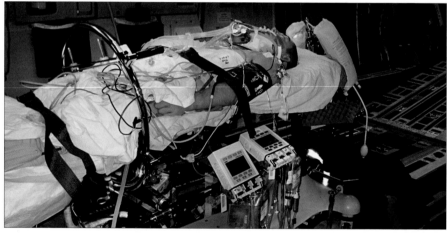

Fig. 6.5 A critically injured casualty is transported aboard a cargo aircraft configured for evacuation. The cargo space affords room for access to the patient or for transport of multiple casualties.

- Very high cost and complexity
- More efficient – medical crew can manage multiple complex casualties
- Possibility of retrograde airlift – use of cargo or passenger airplane to bring supplies to the disaster area and to evacuate casualties as they return for more supplies
- Can only be performed safely with extensive pre-planning and training of the medical crew for challenges of patient loading and

unloading, managing multiple patients inflight, and securing patients and associated medical supplies and equipment.

- A simplified patient care record listing pertinent information (medications, allergies, injuries) facilitates rapid provision of essential care en route.

Patient Stresses of Flight

Hypobaric Environment

- During long-range flight in a passenger or cargo aircraft, the actual altitude is typically 30,000-40,000 ft. Cabin altitude is often 5,000 to 8,000 ft, but can be higher.

    o According to Boyle's Law, gas volume is inversely proportional to pressure at a constant temperature.

    o At a cabin altitude of 8,000 ft, a gas bubble will increase in volume by a factor of 1.35 compared with the volume at sea level.

    o If there is a loss of cabin pressure at 34,000 ft, the factor for gas expansion becomes 4.04.

- **Trapped gas in any body cavity can cause serious consequences as it expands on ascent.**

- Special attention must be paid to trapped gas within the thorax, cranium, eye, middle ear, paranasal sinuses, and the gut in the presence of an ileus.

- Patient care appliances are also susceptible to this effect, particularly endotracheal tube cuffs, pulmonary artery catheter balloons, pressure bags for intravenous fluids, and mechanical ventilators, which may require recalibration at altitude.

- The decreased ambient pressure also affects edema formation through a decrease in Starling forces.

    o Casualties with decreased oncotic pressure or increased vascular permeability are particularly susceptible to this.

    o The consequences are potentially serious in patients with impending compartment syndrome in the extremities or abdomen.

- Achieving a lower cabin altitude requires flying at a lower altitude, which is not always practical.

    o This increases fuel consumption, which decreases aircraft range.

    o It may expose the flight to more turbulence.

    o It may not be possible, depending on the terrain the mission has to fly over.

CASE VIGNETTE

The victims of a bombing incident were evacuated by air. Many of the victims had no clinically apparent lung abnormality at sea level, but developed significant oxyhemoglobin desaturation in-flight due to occult blast injury. These casualties required supplemental oxygen, resulting in greater than expected consumption of oxygen supplies on the aircraft.

Decreased Partial Pressure of Oxygen

- **The partial pressure of oxygen in the ambient air decreases with increasing altitude.**

    o At a cabin altitude of 8,000 feet, the barometric pressure is 565 mm Hg and arterial PO_2 for normal individuals is in the range of 55-60 mm Hg.

    o Casualties with impaired gas exchange will experience hypoxemia on exposure to this altitude, the degree of which is difficult to predict.

- Monitor patients in-flight with pulse oximetry or arterial blood gas analysis and be prepared to provide supplemental oxygen.

    o It is difficult to predict the degree of supplemental oxygen that will be required due to individual differences in respiratory pattern and lung pathology.

    o Titrate supplemental oxygen to a meaningful clinical or physiologic endpoint.

Acceleration/G-forces

- **Takeoffs and landings present unique challenges.** Litter casualties in large cargo aircraft are typically loaded in alignment with the long axis of the aircraft. As a result, during takeoff and landing recumbent litter patients are exposed to significant acceleration forces along the long axis of their body. This acceleration can result in brief, but significant, intravascular fluid shifts and changes in intracranial pressure.

- An important element of pre-mission planning is to coordinate with the flight crew to understand whether the planned flight profile presents any significant physiologic issues and, if so, how they can be modified.

- Acceleration during takeoff is generally not modifiable without affecting flight safety.

- During landing, pilots sometimes decelerate rapidly so they can use a cross-taxiway to save time and fuel and to clear the active runway. In many cases, the pilot can decelerate more slowly by using the entire runway, thus minimizing the physiologic effect of deceleration.

- Elevating the casualty's head, when appropriate, can decrease these effects because the force vector along the patient's long axis will be decreased, resulting in less hemodynamic effect. Some litters are constructed to permit this. On others, this can be accomplished using pillows or blankets. Elevating the casualty's head excessively is unsafe if it prevents adequately securing him/her to the litter.

RISK ALERT!

If a casualty with an unstable cardiac status and fluid overload is positioned head-to-rear during takeoff, the acceleration will cause an acute increase in central venous pressure and worsen fluid overload.

Ascent/Descent

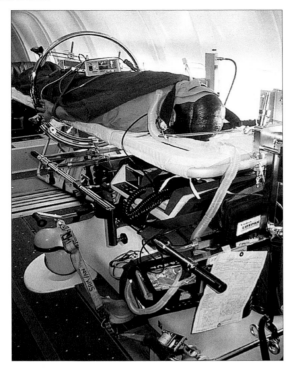

Fig. 6.6 A spinal immobilization bed has been adapted for use during air evacuation.

- The angle of the aircraft relative to horizontal during ascent and descent alters patient physiology in the same way that the Trendelenburg and reverse-Trendelenburg positions do while on land. This effect is less dramatic than the acceleration/deceleration during takeoff and landing, but the effect can last for 10-30 minutes.

- The angle during ascent/descent varies depending on the aircraft model and the flight profile.

- The flight profile is potentially modifiable in coordination with the aircrew and air traffic control, but the physiologic benefits of this must be balanced against safety-of-flight concerns of deviating from established approach/departure routes.

- Decisions on how to position the patient relative to horizontal are the same as those in the terrestrial Intensive Care Unit (ICU).

Turbulence

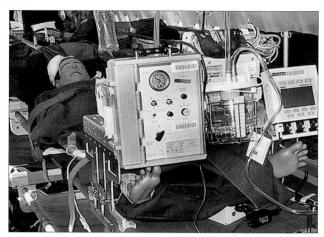

Fig. 6.7 A bracket has been developed that secures to a standard litter and allows optimal positioning of medical equipment.

- Avoiding turbulence during long-range air evacuation is often impossible for the aircrew, and turbulence can occur abruptly. The medical crew needs to plan each mission as if significant turbulence will occur and consider how it will affect both medical gear and the patient.
- The casualties at greatest risk from turbulence are those with unstable fractures, particularly spinal instability.

    o Spinal immobilization beds have been adapted for use during air evacuation and are reliable and easy to use.

    o External fixators are a reliable way to immobilize extremity fractures during evacuation.

    o Traction with hanging weights cannot be used during air evacuation because of their susceptibility to acceleration and turbulence, but traction can be provided with calibrated springs.

- Medical supplies and equipment that are not secure during turbulence can become projectiles, creating a hazard in the aircraft and rendering the gear inoperable.
- Medical devices in use on a patient must be secured in a way that provides the medical crew with adequate access to read the displays and adjust the controls.
- Special roll-pack bags can be secured along the fuselage of some aircraft. The bags can be unrolled, giving rapid access to the contents of the bag's pockets.
- Pocketed-vests or waist-packs can be used to give immediate access to small items needed frequently during the transport.

Vibration

- Casualties and crew are exposed to varying degrees of vibration during long-range air transport. This vibration can cause patients increased wound pain, particularly in the case of orthopedic fractures. Padding fractured extremities can minimize this.

- Vibration also causes casualties and medical crew to fatigue more rapidly than on the ground. This should be factored into planning for long or multiple evacuations on a vibration-prone aircraft. In general, rotary-wing and propeller-driven aircraft vibrate more than jet aircraft.

Temperature Control

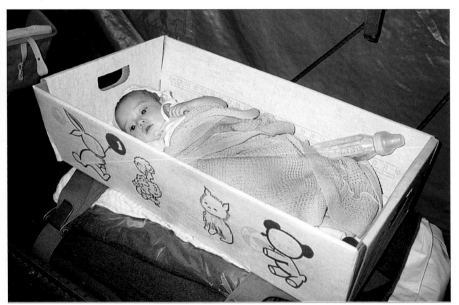

RISK ALERT!

The casualties who are most susceptible to irregular temperature control are post-surgical patients, young children, and those with burns.

Fig. 6.8 Orange crate doubles as pediatric evacuation stretcher, El Salvador earthquake (1987)

- Tight temperature control in the cabin of a cargo aircraft is often difficult to achieve. The aircraft ventilation system can create locations within the cabin that are consistently either too hot or too cold.

- Consult with the aircrew before and during the mission to meet the patient's temperature requirements.

- Young children, burn victims, and post-surgical casualties are particularly susceptible to temperature changes.

Humidity

- The ambient humidity of cabin air during high-altitude flight is extremely low, generally below 5-10%.

- The medical crew needs to factor this in to estimate insensible water loss, particularly in burn casualties.

- Respiratory secretions can become dangerously viscous, especially with tracheotomies, unless the casualties are breathing humidified oxygen.

Noise

- Cargo aircraft often lack the soundproofing found in commercial airliners. The constant noise in these aircraft results in increased fatigue, interferes with communication, prevents useful patient auscultation, and presents a long-term occupational risk of hearing loss for the medical crew.

Clinical Capability in Fixed-Wing Evacuation

Given current technology, many of the aspects of ground-based medical care can be replicated during evacuation.

- Life-saving procedures – small kits are available for the performance of:

    o Airway management – endotracheal intubation, laryngeal mask airway, cricothyrotomy

    o Vascular access – central line, cut-down, or intraosseous infusion

    o Thoracostomy – tube or catheter

- Physiologic monitoring, including electrocardiogram, pulse oximetry, non-invasive and invasive pressure monitoring, and capnometry

- Mechanical ventilation

- Cardiac pacing and defibrillation

- Diagnostic electrocardiography

- Infusion pumps

- Laboratory analyzer – for basic serum chemistry and hematologic testing and arterial blood gas analysis

TREATMENT ALERT!

Infusion pumps are critical in controlling the rate of vasoactive infusions in air evacuation. The effects of barometric pressure change on trapped gas make gravity-based systems for controlling drip rate unreliable during air evacuation.

Certain features of medical equipment are required for their safe use during evacuation:

- Small size – due to space constraints.

- Adequate battery life – to permit operation during breaks in access to electrical power that can occur during evacuation.

- Airworthiness – the equipment must have been demonstrated to function under conditions of altitude, vibration, acceleration, heat, and cold.

- Electromagnetic testing – must demonstrate that emissions from the equipment will not interfere with aircraft systems, and that emissions from the aircraft will not cause malfunction of the medical device. Electromagnetic interference from medical equipment has been implicated in fatal aircraft accidents.

Oxygen storage is a special challenge in air evacuation. Oxygen is hazardous cargo that presents significant safety-of-flight concerns. There are two major forms of oxygen storage used in air evacuation:

- Compressed gas offers the advantages of availability, simplicity, and stability in storage. Ensuring the security of gas cylinders is critical, both when moving the cylinders on and off the aircraft and during flight. A cylinder that is damaged can become a projectile. Another disadvantage is the relatively high weight and volume of the cylinders required to provide large quantities of oxygen.

- Liquid oxygen (LOX) converters change stored liquid oxygen to gas. LOX storage is built into some aircraft. LOX offers advantages over compressed gas in terms of weight and volume. One liter of LOX converts to approximately 800 liters of gaseous oxygen. LOX is also free of the risk of explosive decompression of a ruptured, compressed gas cylinder. However, it may be difficult to obtain the resources needed to recharge LOX converters at the disaster scene.

- Available systems can generate oxygen from a solid state. These are useful for emergency oxygen supplies for crew and passengers, but are not yet practical for the large volumes of oxygen required for medical use.

Casualty Preparation

Preparation begins with identifying which casualties should be evacuated and planning the logistics of the evacuation. This includes the timing and mode of evacuation, clinical preparation, special medical personnel and equipment requirements, and their destination facility.

- Casualties evacuated from a disaster area may be distributed to multiple receiving facilities and become separated from relatives.

- Evacuations should be tracked by logging patient names and basic clinical information to facilitate reuniting family members who are separated during the event.

- At a minimum, logging patient demographics will facilitate reunion.

- Pre-numbered cards that produce multiple copies using simple methods, such as carbon paper, allow the sending medical team, transport team, and receiving medical team to have a consistent chain of identification.

Clinical Preparation

Useful planning tools before the mission include a systematic review of the stresses of flight, with consideration of how they will apply to each casualty, and brainstorming of possible complications that can arise during evacuation and how best to address them. Specific items that bear mention are:

- **Oxygen therapy**—consider giving supplemental oxygen to patients with known hypoxemia, dyspnea, or anemia. Ensuring an adequate oxygen supply is critical. The table at the end of this chapter presents the steps for oxygen calculation for a single casualty.

- **Mechanical ventilation**—steps must be taken to reduce the risk of tracheal injury and/or endotracheal (ET) tube cuff rupture from expansion of the cuff at altitude.

  o The air can be removed from the cuff and replaced by Normal Saline solution with sufficient pressure to eliminate leakage around the cuff.

  o If the medical crew is equipped with a cuff manometer, this can be used with an air-filled cuff to monitor and adjust cuff pressure during ascent and descent.

- **Trapped gas**—in general, all trapped gas should be evacuated before long-range transport by air to eliminate the risk of tissue damage from gas expansion.

o **Pneumothorax**—a functioning chest tube should be in place with a Heimlich valve in line in case the pleural drainage unit must be rapidly disconnected for emergency exit.

o **Ileus**—recent abdominal surgery is not a contraindication to air transport, but if the casualty has an ileus, a functioning nasogastric tube must be secured and attached to suction.

o **Obstructed middle ear and paranasal sinuses**—this can be assessed by the patient's response to the Valsalva maneuver. If obstruction is present, it can generally be managed by application of a topical vasoconstrictor such as oxymetazoline.

o **Intra-ocular/intracranial air**—casualties with trapped intra-ocular/intracranial air should not be airlifted unless the risk of not being evacuated outweighs the risk of complications from gas expansion, potentially causing retinal ischemia or increased intracranial pressure and herniation. This risk is related to the volume of trapped gas and whether or not the gas has any means to vent with expansion.

o **Cabin altitude restriction**—should be considered in all of the above situations if the trapped gas cannot be relieved.

- **Decompression sickness/arterial gas embolism**—casualties with these conditions should not be exposed to altitudes greater than that of the origination airfield.

    o Portable recompression chambers have been developed and are the ideal solution to this problem.

    o Casualties can also be managed with the highest concentration of oxygen available as a means of washing out body nitrogen stores and decreasing bubble size. Ideally, 100% oxygen should be administered through a closed system with a tight-fitting mask to permit administration of oxygen without inhaling further environmental nitrogen.

- **Casts**—casualties are prone to edema formation on exposure to altitude, and this risk increases with damaged tissue and reduced plasma oncotic pressure. This edema can lead to compartment syndrome inside the cast.

    o Casts that have been in place for less than 48-72 hours should be bivalved before evacuation and held closed with elastic dressing if this can be done without compromising fracture stability.

    o If this cannot be done safely, it is imperative to follow the neurovascular status of the limb closely and be prepared to open the cast in-flight if compartment syndrome develops.

- **Abdominal damage control surgery** places casualties at risk for abdominal compartment syndrome with continued volume resuscitation and as edema worsens on exposure to altitude.

    o The medical crew must be prepared to monitor abdominal compartment pressures and open the abdomen if this syndrome develops.

    o If this is not practical, casualties should be transported with their abdomen open.

- **Burns** place patients at risk for several flight stresses, including impaired thermoregulation, increased insensible fluid loss, and difficult infection control.

    o Blankets, sleeping bags, heat-conserving dressings, and/or active warming devices should be used to prevent hypothermia.

    o Wounds should be dressed immediately pre-flight and not undressed in-flight if at all possible, to reduce the risk of contamination from the environment.

    o Strong consideration should be given to performing endotracheal intubation pre-flight in patients with significant inhalation injury. It is difficult to monitor the airway and to perform intubation in-flight.

- **Violent/psychotic patients** present a risk to themselves and to flight safety during air evacuation.

    o Plan for adequate restraint and sedation.

    o Some casualties may require their own medical attendant to closely monitor their behavior and intervene rapidly if required.

- **Infection control** is a special challenge during air evacuation. Patients with known or suspected infections requiring respiratory isolation should not be transported by air unless essential. If these patients are moved, several factors should be considered:

    o Discuss isolation requirements and appropriate airflow pattern within the cabin.

    o Ensure the use of proper isolation masks by the patient and all other personnel aboard the aircraft.

    o Carry adequate quantities of isolation supplies and take steps to control secretions, such as diarrhea, if patients require contact isolation.

Oxygen Calculation Requirements

Courtesy of US Air Force

Step 1: Oxygen Requirement				
Patient Oxygen Usage Rate $\frac{(FiO_2 - 0.21)}{0.79}$	X	Minute Volume	=	Required Liters Per Minute (LPM)
Flight duration	+	Ground time	=	Mission duration
Required Liters Per Minute (LPM)	X	60	=	Required Liters Per Hour (LPH)
Mission duration	X	Required LPH	=	**Total oxygen requirements**

Step 2: Oxygen Supply				
Compressed oxygen *Tank pressure (psi)*	X	Tank factor #	=	Available volume (gaseous liters)
Liquid Oxygen *Liquid liters*	X	804	=	Available volume (gaseous liters)

Step 3: Does supply exceed requirement by safety factor?*

# Tank factors	Cylinder Size	Tank Factor
	D	0.16
	E	0.28
	Q	0.94
	M	1.56
	G	2.41
	H	3.14

*Safety factor: Determine quantity of excess oxygen to carry based on specific mission parameters such as weather and likelihood of diversion. A 2-hour excess is a reasonable safety factor in the absence of special circumstances.

PATIENT SUMMARY CARD

(PATIENT CARE TRANSPORT SUMMARY)

NAME_____

DOB _____ M / F _____

ORIGINATING LOCATION _____

DESTINATION_____

ALLERGIES_____

MEDICATION	DOSE	ROUTE	TIME

INJURIES/INTERVENTIONS

_____

_____

_____

_____

_____

POTENTIAL TRANSPORT COMPLICATIONS _____

_____

_____

_____

Summary

Evacuation is an important, but often neglected, aspect of disaster preparedness. Evacuation of injured disaster victims requires knowledge of the unique patient stresses of flight and adequate preparation to meet these challenges to ensure patient safety during evacuation.

KEY POINTS

 Important patient stresses of flight include the hypobaric environment and decreased partial pressure of oxygen encountered with increasing altitude.

 Indications for evacuation include: decompression of the disaster area, improving care for critical patients and providing care for specific high-risk injuries such as blast injuries, crush injuries, and burns.

 Disaster planning must include realistic planning for evacuation of casualties.

Public Health Priorities

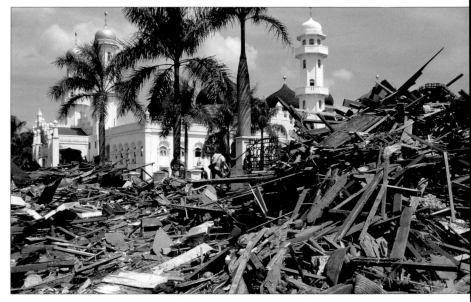

Fig. 7.1 Tsunami, Indonesia (2004)

CASE SCENARIO

In 2004, a devastating tsunami affected many countries abutting the Indian Ocean, including Indonesia. The epicenter was located off the west coast of Sumatra, Indonesia. One of the most severely impacted regions was Banda Aceh, an area affected by pre-disaster war and poverty, making emergency relief a challenge for all the responding international organizations. The Rapid Needs Assessment (RNA) was a valuable technique to assess the disaster's impact on the community's public health and medical services.

Introduction

Disasters pose significant challenges to the communities they impact. Public health and medical services are often disrupted by the physical damage and overwhelmed by an increased patient load. Since the healthcare infrastructure is an integral component of the overall response, a rapid and accurate assessment of the impact is essential to a swift and effective recovery. Responders must understand the magnitude of the incident, the resources available to provide temporary restoration of public health and medical services, and the priorities for recovery.

The challenges related to this task are twofold:

- The needs assessment must be performed concurrently with the provision of emergency health services.
- Planning the response will be based by necessity on limited assessment information.

The key in resolving this dilemma is in the pre-planning phase of disaster response. Responders should develop and exercise their capacity to perform needs assessments. This challenge is somewhat mitigated by the requirement to establish adequate lifeline services as a priority. Potable water, safe food of good quality and sufficient quantity, effective sanitation, adequate living space, and an environment free of threats are absolute necessities that must be addressed as first priorities.

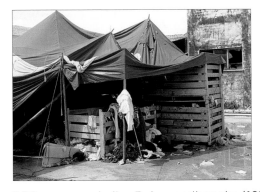

Fig. 7.2 Temporary shelter, Turkey earthquake (1999)

One technique used to assess the disaster's impact on the community's public health and medical services is the RNA. Use of new technologies can greatly support the performing aspects of the RNA. Recent technologic advances in global positioning and social media have enabled responders to access information previously unavailable in the disaster setting. These advances enable responders to organize and analyze information as maps, checklists, and charts in real-time in the field setting.

Cardinal Questions of a Rapid Needs Assessment (RNA)

1. What are the health and medical consequences of the event?
2. Are there infrastructure problems/potential problems regarding:
   a. Health and medical
      - Immediate life-threatening injuries/illnesses
      - Epidemic and endemic diseases
      - Disrupted/overwhelmed services
   b. Potable water: quality and quantity
   c. Food: quality and quantity
   d. Shelter
   e. Sanitation
   f. Mental health
   g. Physical safety in the shelter areas
3. Is the local community able to respond?
4. How is the community communicating?

The Rapid Needs Assessment (RNA)

The RNA provides a timely evaluation of the impact of a disaster on the public health and medical infrastructure in an affected population.

Assessment information can be obtained from a variety of sources:

- Existing information collection systems, e.g., public health surveillance systems
- Relief worker/first-responder reports
- Conventional media reports
- Social media reports

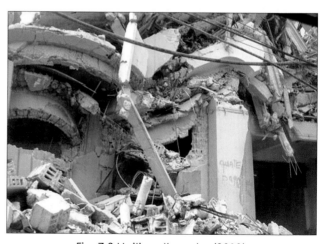

Fig. 7.3 Haiti earthquake (2010)

FIELD TIP

Media reports often provide overview information regarding the magnitude of a disaster, particularly in the areas of greatest impact. Their ability to gain firsthand observational information through use of helicopters and on-scene reporters can provide visual information that can be used to estimate greatest damage and impact.

The specific elements of the RNA are as follows:

1. Determine the overall magnitude of the event.
2. Determine the disruption of lifeline services.
3. Determine the extent of the local response and the impact on the health and medical systems.

Element 1: Assessing the Magnitude of a Disaster

Much information about the impact of the disaster can be obtained prior to arriving onsite, from news reports and telephone communication. Once on-site, discussions with health officials, rescue workers, and others can quickly provide details about the severity of the event and the areas of most severe impact.

Responders performing the RNA may face challenges in trying to determine the magnitude of the disaster. Downed power lines, blocked-off roads, police barricades, and continued threats to physical well-being can prevent responders from gaining access to large areas. Visual assessment by air is often the best method. Using a grid approach, pilots can fly over affected areas and plot the levels of relative damage on maps.

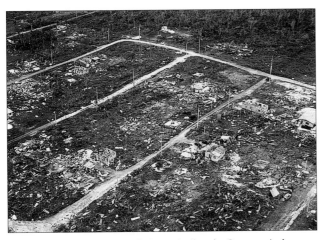

Fig. 7.4 Aerial view of devastation in Guam during Supertyphoon Pongsona (2002)

Element 2: Assessing Lifeline Services

Determining the disruption of lifeline services— potable water supply, sanitation capacity, food supply, shelter, and electricity—is critical to the relief effort. For example, water supply could be disrupted in a number of ways: supply and/or distribution could be interrupted or water could be contaminated.

Lifeline Services: Minimum Requirements

<u>Water</u>

- Drinking: 5 L/day/person
- 15 L/day/person: drinking, cooking, personal hygiene

<u>Food</u>

- Adult: 2,100 kcal/person/day
- Children: varies by age

<u>Emergency/Temporary Shelter</u>

- 3.5 m²/person

(Sphere Standards)

Element 3: Assessing the Local Response

The extent to which the local public health and medical community is responding to the demands of the disaster has a direct bearing on the deployment of resources from the outside. The assessment can include evaluation of:

- The emergency medical services system (EMS)
- The hospital system
- Pharmacy services
- Public health clinic schedules
- The capacity to sustain medical response over time
- Health status indicators
- Mental health indicators such as reports of domestic violence and substance abuse
- Other health and medical indicators that provide information about the local response

Standard of Practice: Health Status Indicators

Pre-disaster baseline information on the health of a community is important in defining the magnitude of the disaster. Changes from baseline can be used to measure a disaster's impact.

Mortality
- Deaths resulting from event
- Deaths per location
- Deaths by specific population subset, e.g., children, elderly

Morbidity
- Injuries
    - o Types (upper/lower extremity; blunt/penetrating)
    - o Subset of population (male/female; adult/child)

Illness
- Types—communicable, epidemic
- Facility/Service
    - o EMS runs
    - o Hospital capacity
    - o Emergency department visits
    - o Mental health visits

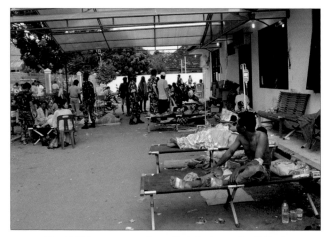

Fig. 7.5 Temporary hospital, Indonesia (2004)

Conducting the RNA

There are several steps in conducting an RNA. Since initial disaster response efforts are directed toward saving lives and preventing disease, the initial steps of an RNA are directed at identifying what is needed to achieve those goals. The areas that the RNA must address are described in the box below.

Standard of Practice: The Public Health RNA

1. Nature of the Event
   - Area affected
   - Damage severity
   - Estimated fatalities
   - Ongoing risks
   - Predicted weather conditions
2. Size of the Community Affected
   - Populations displaced
3. Community Resources Prior to the Event
   - Community resources and infrastructure
   - Public transportation
   - Radio/television
4. Healthcare Impact
   - Numbers of injured/ill
   - Damage to the hospital facilities, personnel, supplies, including hospitals on generator power
   - Damage to EMS, including dispatch capacity
   - Damage to clinics/pharmacies/dialysis facilities
   - Public health infrastructure (surveillance, immunization)

Standard of Practice: The Public Health RNA (*Cont*)

5. Water
- Status of current water supply
- Status of current water distribution system
- Sources of potable water
- Water-testing system status
- Sanitation systems status

6. Food
- Adequacy of food supply
- Perishable foods storage
- Sources of food
- Potential for malnutrition

7. Shelter
- Significant damage to residential areas
- Extent of need for temporary shelter
- Supply of existing safe, well-stocked shelters
- Predicted weather for the next 7 days
- Significant electricity outages

Surveillance

Use of pre-existing functional surveillance systems within the community is recommended as a way of obtaining baseline community information and initial epidemiologic information. Surveillance activities should be utilized to assess specific issues, such as the scope of post-disaster health consequences, vulnerable populations, emerging diseases, and intervention assessments. Particular attention should be placed on vulnerable populations such as infants, children, pregnant women, and the elderly. These groups can be more susceptible to infectious diseases, inadequate nutrition, and stresses associated with environmental hazards commonly seen after disasters.

Sample Active Surveillance Report

Healthcare Facility/Team _____

Reporting Period: Time/Date _____ to Time/Date _____

Cases	<15 years of age	≥15 years of age
Fever		
Fever with diarrhea		
Cough with fever		
Rash		
Meningitis		
Injury		
Death		
Comments:		

Challenges in Conducting an RNA

There are challenges to obtaining the necessary information to develop an accurate needs assessment:

- Blocked access or restricted travel to the affected areas
- Ongoing physical danger to responders

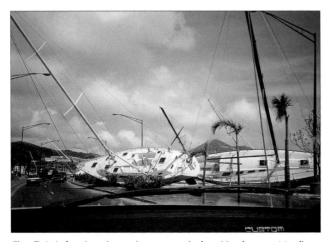

Fig. 7.6 Infrastructure damage during Hurricane Marilyn, St. Thomas, Virgin Islands (1995)

A case definition is a standardized symptom complex.

- Inaccessible or destroyed records for baseline analysis
- Lack of "denominator data," e.g., post-disaster changes in population
- Under-reporting of disease
- Poor sampling techniques
- Non-standardized reporting/case definitions

Final Reporting

The results of the RNA need to be reported to the appropriate local community response organizers. The RNA report should be written in a concise format stating the sources of information used, the infrastructure sectors evaluated, the problems identified, and the suggested recommendations to address the needs and processes necessary to identify future problems. The RNA can also be used to monitor the progress of the response and in determining the point at which assistance is no longer necessary.

Summary

Timely surveillance systems and rapid needs assessments are required to fully evaluate the effects of a disaster on the public health and medical systems of the impacted region. These activities are needed not only in the immediate disaster area but also in areas that house displaced persons outside of the disaster area. It is critical to recognize that the medical response to disasters depends on non-medical elements that provide essential infrastructure (food, water, shelter, sanitation, security, transportation, communication, and supplies).

KEY POINTS

 The rapid needs assessment often must be performed concurrently with the delivery of emergency health services.

 Potable water, safe food, effective sanitation, temporary housing, and an environment free of threats are key first priorities in disaster response.

 Social media is increasingly important as a means of communication in disasters, especially in austere environments.

Disaster Risk Management

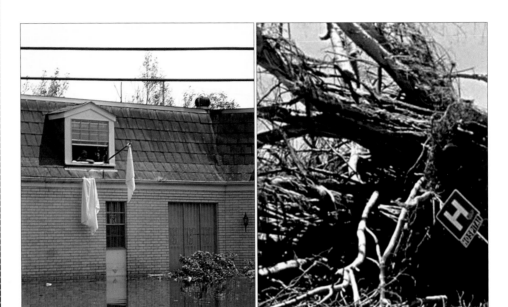

Figs. 8.1, 8.2 Hurricane Katrina, New Orleans (2005)

CASE SCENARIO

Hurricane Katrina was one of the most expensive and devastating hurricanes in the history of the United States. Beginning on August 23, 2005 in the Bahamas, Hurricane Katrina impacted much of the Gulf Coast in the United States. Within the span of one month, Hurricane Katrina devastated thousands of miles of the Gulf coastline.

The City of New Orleans in Louisiana sustained extensive damage, both from the hurricane and from multiple breaches to the levees. Significant flooding of the entire City of New Orleans occurred and forced the closing of all medical facilities in the city, requiring evacuation of all hospitalized patients to mobile and fixed facilities outside the affected areas. In addition to the significant mortality (deaths) and morbidity (injuries) caused by the hurricane and levee breeches, the City of New Orleans sustained overwhelming economic and environmental losses that exceeded the ability of the affected communities to cope using their own resources.

Introduction

A disaster is "a serious disruption of the functioning of a community or a society causing widespread human, material, economic or environmental losses that exceed the ability of the affected community or society to cope using its own resources" (United Nationals International Strategy for Disaster Reduction [UNISDR] 2009).

An event that does not exceed a community or society's capacity to cope is classified as an emergency rather than a disaster (World Health Organization [WHO], 1998). Emergencies and disasters are thus part of a relative continuum of events that differ only by the degree of severity. **Risk reduction actions reduce the number of events that exceed the community or society's ability to respond, thereby preventing some emergencies from ever becoming disasters.**

Disaster consequences may include loss of life, injury, disease, and other negative effects on human physical, mental, and social well-being, together with damage to property, destruction of assets, loss of services, social and economic disruption and environmental degradation (UNISDR, 2009). The severity of these consequences is referred to as disaster impact. Disasters occur as a result of the combination of three factors:

- Population exposure to a hazard
- The conditions of vulnerability that are present
- Insufficient capacity or measures to reduce or cope with the potential negative consequences.

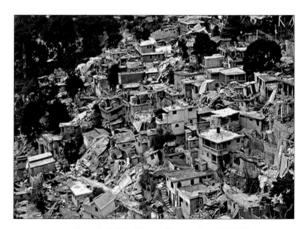

Fig. 8.3 Haiti earthquake (2010)

Risk is defined as the probability of harmful consequences or expected losses resulting from interactions between natural or human-induced hazards and vulnerable conditions (UNISDR, 2009). These consequences could occur in a particular community or society over some specified future period.

> **DISASTER RISK =**
> **HAZARD x POPULATION VULNERABILITY – ABSORPTIVE CAPACITY**

The disaster risk equation has been applied to estimate disaster risk according to the following relationship: $p(D) = k[p(H) \times p(V)] - AC$.

- $p(D)$ = risk of disaster impact
- $p(H)$ = the probability of hazard occurrence
- $p(V)$ = the probability of population vulnerability
- AC = absorptive capacity (also known as adaptive capacity).

According to this equation, disaster risk may be reduced among populations at risk by reducing the hazard itself, by decreasing the vulnerability, and by increasing the absorptive capacity.

Absorptive capacity and resilience are not synonymous. *Resilience* is the *ability* of a system, community, or society exposed to hazards to resist, absorb, accommodate, and recover from the effects of a hazard in a timely and efficient manner through the preservation and restoration of its essential basic structures and functions. **Resilience** is comprised of:

- Absorbing capacity
- Buffering capacity
- Response to the event and recovery from the damage sustained

Absorptive capacity **is the limit of this overall ability.**

For any hazard, risk varies with the following factors related to the disaster (D):

- Vulnerability of the population (the degree of population susceptibility (S)
- Exposure (E)
- Resilience (R)

Disaster Risk

Risk management is activity directed toward assessing, controlling, and monitoring risks. Strategies for risk management include risk assessment and control measures. These control measures in turn include transferring the risk to another party, avoiding the risk, reducing the negative effect of the risk, and accepting some or all of the consequences of a particular risk. ISO 31000 is a set of international standards relating to risk management recently codified by the International Organization for Standardization (2009).

Disaster risk management applies the general principles of risk management to disasters. Figure 1 and Table 1 describe the components of disaster risk management, including both assessment and control.

The process for disaster risk management

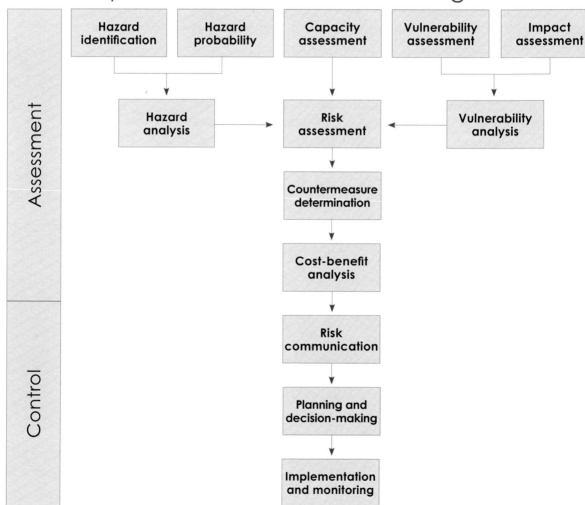

Figure 1: Schematic overview of the process for risk management

Component	Activities
Hazard Analysis • Hazard identification • Hazard probability	Identifying hazards with the potential to cause loss or damage of an asset Determining frequency of past hazard events
Impact Assessment • Asset assessment • Loss assessment	Determining critical assets (e.g., population, medical facilities, etc.) Identifying expected loss or damage of each asset for each hazard Prioritizing assets based on consequence of loss
Capacity Assessment	Identifying strengths, attributes, and resources available to respond and recover from a disaster
Vulnerability Assessment • Exposure • Susceptibility	Estimating degree of vulnerability of each asset for each hazard Identifying pre-existing countermeasures and their level of effectiveness
Countermeasure Determination • Avoidance / reduction • Transfer / retention	Identifying new countermeasures that may be taken to eliminate or lessen hazards and/or vulnerabilities
Cost - Benefit Analysis	Identifying countermeasure costs and benefits Prioritizing options
Risk Communication	Preparing a range of recommendations for decision-makers and/or the public
Risk Management Plan	A plan for disaster risk treatment is developed for each phase of the emergency cycle.
Implementation and Monitoring	The risk management program is implemented and monitored according to plan.

Table 1: Key components of disaster risk management (Adapted from Keim, 2002)

Disaster risk management is a comprehensive all-hazards approach that entails developing and implementing strategies for each phase of the disaster life cycle. Disaster risk management includes both pre-impact and post-impact disaster risk reduction:

- **Pre-impact:** prevention, preparedness, and mitigation
- **Post-impact:** disaster risk retention (response and recovery).

Disaster Life Cycle

The emphasis on a "life-cycle" approach to risk management is important in the case of disasters. **All disasters follow a cyclical pattern known as the disaster life cycle, which includes five stages: prevention, mitigation, preparedness, response, and recovery.** These phases often overlap each other in time and in scope. The underlying drive of disaster management is to reduce risk both to human life and to systems important to livelihood.

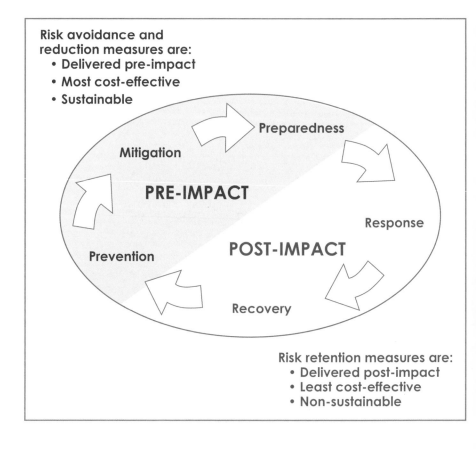

Figure 2 depicts the process of risk management as applied to the disaster cycle. It compares risk avoidance and reduction measures (in the upper left) to risk retention measures (in the lower right).

This depiction of disasters as cyclical in nature may seem to imply that disasters are inevitable. This is not the case. **The goals of risk avoidance and risk reduction are to avert disasters and retained risk.**

Risk Assessment

Ideally, disaster risk management is based on a prioritization process. Once risks have been identified, they are assessed in terms of the potential severity of loss and to the probability of occurrence. The risks with the greatest loss and the greatest probability of occurrence are handled first, and risks with lower loss and lower probability of occurrence are handled in descending order. In practice, the process can be very difficult.

A fundamental difficulty in disaster risk assessment is determining the probability of occurrence since statistical information is not available on many kinds of incidents. Furthermore, evaluating the severity of the consequences (impact) is often difficult. Outcomes such as mental illness are difficult to quantify. Thus, expert opinion and available statistics are the primary sources of information. Nevertheless, risk assessment can produce useful information that clarifies risks and helps support decisions.

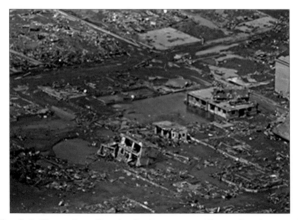

Fig. 8.4 Complex disaster in Japan: earthquake, tsunami, and nuclear reactor meltdown (2011)

Risk Management

Once risks have been identified and assessed, techniques to manage the risk fall into one or more of these four major categories:

- Avoidance (eliminate)
- Reduction (mitigate)
- Transfer (outsource or insure)
- Retention (accept and budget)

Table 2 compares the four major categories of risk reduction to: the three stages of prevention; the five phases of the disaster cycle; and the three major components of disaster risk management. It can be seen that these various stages are complementary and can be combined to create a unified approach to the management of disaster risk.

Stage of Prevention	Phase of emergency management cycle		Risk management technique	Disaster risk management component
Primary prevention	Prevention		Risk avoidance	Hazard avoidance
Secondary prevention	Preparedness (susceptibility / resilience)		Risk reduction	Vulnerability reduction
	Mitigation	Structural (exposure)		
		Financial (susceptibility / resilience)	Risk transfer	
Tertiary prevention	Response		Risk retention	Residual risk
	Recovery			

Table 2: A comparison among various techniques for prevention, emergency management, and risk management as applied to disasters

Disaster Risk Avoidance

While people may not always have the ability to prevent disasters from occurring, the health sector can play an important role in preventing the public health impact. The risk of a public health disaster occurs when vulnerable populations are both exposed and susceptible to environmental hazards. Primary prevention seeks to prevent the hazard exposure from occurring. This function is consistent with the category of risk management known as risk avoidance. Examples include land use zoning and regulations that prevent settlement in disaster-prone areas like floodplains. The role of public health in disaster risk avoidance is largely one of scientific leadership (identifying risk factors for morbidity and mortality and advocacy for healthy people, healthy homes, healthy communities, and healthy commerce that are free from disaster risk).

Disaster Risk Reduction

Disaster reduction has emerged as a core element of sustainable development. The 2002 World Summit on Sustainable Development (WSSD) concluded that **"An integrated multi-hazard, inclusive approach to address vulnerability, risk assessment, and disaster management, including prevention, mitigation, preparedness, response, and recovery, is an essential part of a safer world in the twenty-first century."** Reducing risk requires long-term engagement in the development process, and the actual work of disaster risk reduction is largely a task for local personnel.

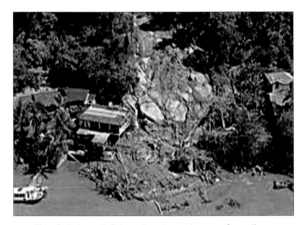

Fig. 8.5 Landslides due to extreme flooding, Brazil (2011)

Risk reduction involves methods that reduce the severity of the loss or the likelihood of the loss from occurring. Secondary prevention aims to detect the disaster hazard event early to control its advance and reduce the resulting health burden. Risk reduction activities seek to prepare for and mitigate the health consequences of disasters that cannot be prevented.

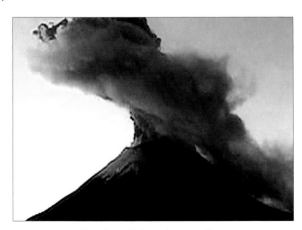

Fig. 8.6 Volcanic eruption

Risk retention involves accepting disaster loss when it occurs and then attempting to respond and recover, if possible. All residual risks that are not avoided or transferred are retained by default. Tertiary prevention seeks to prevent additional risk once the adverse event has occurred. This stage of prevention aims to reduce morbidity, avoid complications, and restore function. Examples of risk retention activities include the provision of medical care or temporary shelter to disaster-affected populations. Risk retention corresponds well to the disaster-cycle phases of response and recovery.

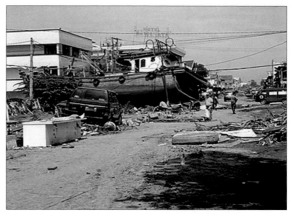

Fig. 8.7 Tsunami, Indonesia (2005)

A disaster risk management plan selects appropriate controls or countermeasures to manage each risk. An effective risk management plan should include a schedule for control implementation and persons responsible for those actions. **Risk communication is a key part of the disaster risk management plan.**

Risk Management for Health

Disaster risk reduction shares some tenets with preventive medicine. As in preventive medicine, risk reduction calls for a basic attitude shift in the minds of many who traditionally get sick first and seek treatment later. When, however, disasters are seen as the outcome of accumulated risk produced by years of vulnerability and underlying hazards, the case for preventive action can be made more plainly. **The challenge for disaster risk reduction as applied to health is to broaden the focus of disaster risk management from that of tertiary prevention (response and recovery) to also emphasize primary and secondary prevention (prevention, preparedness, and mitigation).**

Disaster Risk Planning

Public awareness of disaster risk and risk preparation is critical.

Risk communication must be a key part of the disaster risk management plan.

68

The role of the health sector spans across the spectrum of disaster risk reduction to include prevention, mitigation, and preparedness activities. **Disaster risk reduction as applied to health is intended to prevent and/ or reduce the negative health consequences of disaster hazards. This is accomplished by two means:**

- **Hazard avoidance (primary prevention)**
- **Vulnerability reduction (secondary prevention)**

Primary Prevention (Hazard Avoidance)

Primary prevention seeks to prevent adverse events from occurring. Effective management of natural hazards has prevented the risk of numerous disasters caused by floods, cyclones, droughts, and wildfires. For example, floodplain management in areas of frequent flooding may actually prevent flood disasters altogether.

- The primary prevention of disaster risk relies heavily on hazard avoidance through structural measures. These measures include: modification of the physical environment through architectural design, engineering controls, and construction methods and materials in order to prevent hazard exposure. Structural measures for primary prevention are better developed for meteorological (weather-related) disasters than that for geophysical (seismic events) disasters.

- Non-structural measures (e.g., land use strategies, policies and laws, public awareness raising, training, and education) may be the most effective means to prevent many geophysical disaster impacts.

- Hazard monitoring and accurate forecasting, integrated with early warning systems, helps to facilitate the timely initiation of population protection measures that may involve either evacuation or sheltering in place. This is especially true in the case of meteorological hazards (e.g., tornadoes, cyclones, and floods).

Disaster Risk Avoidance

Effective management of natural hazards has prevented the risk of numerous disasters.

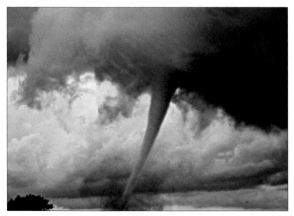

Fig. 8.8 Tornado, Courtesy of NOAA

- Disease surveillance teamed with early warning systems also serve as an effective means for primary prevention of infectious disease disasters.

- Much of the approach to primary prevention of technological disasters is based upon regulation of industrial and commercial practices, including the manufacture, storage, transport, and utilization of hazardous materials as well as the promotion of safe practices in the construction and transportation industries.

Secondary Prevention (Vulnerability Reduction)

Secondary prevention reduces disaster risk by reducing population vulnerability. Human vulnerability to disasters is a complex phenomenon that includes social, economic, health, and cultural factors. Given that a hazard is likely to occur, the risk of a public health disaster is lessened by:

- Reducing human exposures to the hazard by a reduction of human vulnerability.

- Lessening human susceptibility to the hazard.

- Building resilience to the impact of the hazard.

<u>Exposure Reduction</u>

Exposure is defined as subjection to the influence or effects of a disaster-related health hazard. The toxicity or lethality of an environmental health hazard is often characterized by a dose-response relationship. Typically, as the degree of exposure to a health hazard increases, the human emotion of concern—itself an adverse health effect—appears in more of the population. In the case of natural and infectious disease disasters, the degree of exposure of a given population to the hazard (e.g., extremes of wind, temperature, precipitation, seismicity, volcanism, biological agents) has a direct relationship to the incidence and severity of adverse health outcomes. Persons located in close proximity to the disaster hazard have a higher risk for injury and illness as compared with those less exposed. For example, persons living in temperate climate zones may be at higher risk for exposure to hazardous extremes of temperature.

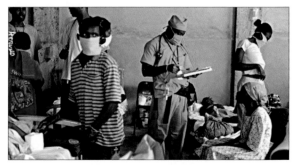

*Fig. 8.9 Cholera outbreak, Haiti (2011),
Courtesy of CDC*

70

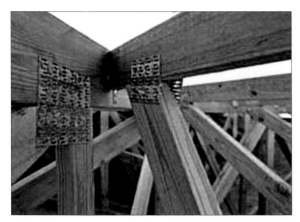

Fig. 8.10 Roof reinforcements, also known as hurricane straps, can mitigate damage done to homes during severe storms, Courtesy of FEMA

Mitigation serves to reduce population vulnerability by reducing population exposure to disaster hazards. **Mitigation may occur as a result of both structural and non-structural measures.** Disaster-related mitigation activities reduce deaths and injuries by reducing exposure of the population to the hazard. Mitigation measures ensure structural safety through enforcement of adequate building codes; promulgating legislation to relocate structures away from disaster-prone areas, land use planning and regulation, and managing high-hazard zones. Critical facilities can be identified before a disaster occurrence, and engineering measures may be taken to mitigate loss of critical health infrastructures and assets during extreme weather events.

While disasters involve the destruction of lives and property, they also create something important: opportunities to improve safety, enhance equity, and rebuild in new or different ways through promotion of "healthy people, healthy homes, and healthy communities." Ideally, those opportunities would be used to produce safer communities with more equitable and sustainable livelihoods for people. Healthy homes are disaster-resilient, designed and built to stay safe during extreme weather events. Healthy communities minimize exposure of people and property to natural disasters. Sustainable communities are disaster-resilient communities.

Susceptibility Reduction

Susceptibility is defined as the likelihood of suffering an adverse health effect when exposed to a given health hazard. Populations are not equally susceptible to the same health hazard. Differences among persons are due to such factors as sex, age, genetic predisposition, and health status. The degree of susceptibility to a given hazard also has a direct relationship to the frequency and severity of adverse health outcomes. Persons more susceptible to a disaster hazard have a higher risk for injury and illness as compared with those less susceptible. For example:

- Elderly persons living in temperate climate zones are more susceptible to heat wave disasters than are young adults living in the same location.
- Vaccinated people are less susceptible to infectious disease disasters.
- Population feeding programs along with de-worming reduce susceptibility to malnutrition and associated co-morbid conditions.

Resilience Building

The resilience of a social system is determined by the degree to which the system has the necessary resources and is capable of organizing itself to develop its capacities to implement disaster risk reduction and to institute means to transfer or manage residual risks. Persons within a population are not equally resilient to the same disaster hazards. Differences among persons are typically due to social and economic factors such as socio-economic status, governmental/organizational structures (e.g., the public health and medical system, social capital, political influence, and behavioral determinants).

The degree of resilience to a given hazard has a direct relationship to the incidence and severity of adverse health outcomes. Persons less resilient to disaster hazards have a higher risk for injury and illness as compared with those who are more resilient. For example, poor, socially isolated, or underprepared persons living in temperate climate zones are less resilient to heat wave disasters than are affluent, well-connected persons who prepare and otherwise ensure their own readiness for such an event. Certain characteristics of the environment may also affect community resilience and make communities more prone or less prone to disasters.

Preparedness implies a behavioral approach focused on actions taken in advance of a disaster in order to reduce its impact. This helps to build resilience from the adverse health effects of disaster hazards. There are other measures besides preparedness that also serve to increase the resilience of a population to disaster hazards. These capacity-building measures may include poverty reduction programs, sustainable development, and social networks that link vulnerable populations together with resources that may assist in the case of disasters. Measures that build surge capacity among human and material resources also help to build disaster resilience.

Tertiary Prevention (Response and Recovery)

<u>Responding to the Public Health Impact of Disasters</u>

Tertiary prevention of disaster risk involves measures taken during the response and recovery phase as a component of risk retention. Disaster response is predominantly focused on immediate and short-term needs and is sometimes called "disaster relief." Response usually includes those actions immediately necessary to remove the affected population from ongoing exposure or risk of harm. Effective response increases the resilience of the population.

Public health is often involved in temporary sheltering and settlement decisions regarding the rapid reinstatement of healthy homes and healthy communities that have a direct impact upon the public health of disaster-affected populations. Public health assists in the delivery of healthcare, performs food safety and water-quality inspections, and assesses sanitation and hygiene in mass care shelters. The demands for environmental health services and consultation are quite high during natural disasters. Public health also becomes involved in health risk assessments and technical assistance related to any suspected hazardous-material exposures after an environmental disaster.

Health communication is a valuable tool in educating the public before and after disaster impact (e.g., protective behaviors that help to prevent drowning or heat illness). Injuries such as electrocutions, burns, and carbon monoxide poisonings are examples of disaster-related morbidity that can be prevented through public awareness and health education.

Health communication is only as effective as it is received and understood by the public. People's understanding of risk is influenced by a host of factors including environment, social ties, culture, and personal prejudices. Warnings do not directly stimulate action, but are processed instead in a personal "risk perception cycle" that is modulated by many factors. The public must be able to:

- **Hear the message**
- **Understand the risk**
- **Believe there is a risk**
- **Believe that the risk can affect them personally**
- **Decide how to respond to the risk**
- **Implement the desired response behavior**

Recovering from the Public Health Impact of Disasters

Rehabilitation and reconstruction begin soon after the emergency phase has ended. Activities should be based on pre-existing strategies and policies that facilitate clear institutional responsibilities for recovery action and enable public participation. The division between the response stage and the subsequent recovery stage is not clear-cut. Some response actions, such as the supply of temporary housing and water supplies, may extend well into the recovery stage.

Recovery programs, coupled with the heightened public awareness after a disaster, also afford a valuable opportunity to develop and implement disaster risk reduction measures and to apply the "build back better" principle. The disaster recovery phase may also offer a window of opportunity for improving risk reduction strategies, such as preparedness and mitigation efforts.

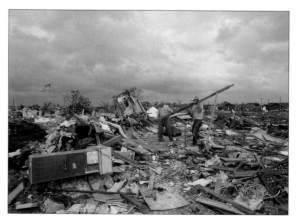

*Fig. 8.11 Tornado damage, Oklahoma, (2013),
Courtesy of FEMA*

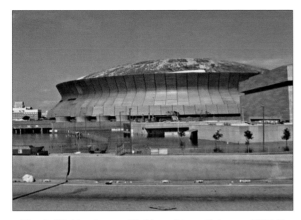

Fig. 8.12 Hurricane Katrina, New Orleans (2005)

Summary

A primary focus on response and recovery is an impractical and inefficient strategy for dealing with disaster threats. Disaster risk management is a comprehensive all-hazard approach that entails developing and implementing strategies for different phases of the disaster life cycle: prevention/mitigation, preparedness, response and recovery, in the context of sustainable development.

Disaster risk management begins with a risk assessment, including an evaluation of hazard frequency and impact as well as the vulnerability of the population and its absorptive capacity to respond to the disaster. This risk assessment is then communicated to stakeholders, and a plan is developed for hazard avoidance (prevention), risk reduction (mitigation and preparedness), and risk retention (response and recovery). Disaster risk management then applies a capability-based approach to treat residual risk not otherwise avoided or transferred.

When disasters are seen as the outcome of accumulated risk produced by years of vulnerability and underlying hazard, the case for preventive action can be made more plainly. **The challenge for disaster risk reduction as applied to health is to broaden the focus of disaster risk management from that of tertiary prevention (response and recovery) to also emphasize primary and secondary prevention (prevention, preparedness, and mitigation).**

KEY POINTS

 Disaster risk management is activity directed toward assessing, controlling, and monitoring risks.

 Disaster risk management is a comprehensive all-hazard approach that entails developing and implementing strategies for each phase of the disaster life cycle (prevention, preparedness, mitigation, response, and recovery).

 Disaster risk reduction shares some attributes with preventive medicine.

 Health communication is a valuable tool in educating the public before and after disaster impact.

The material in this chapter reflects solely the views of the author. It does not necessarily reflect the policies or recommendations of the Centers for Disease Control and Prevention or the U.S. Department of Health and Human Services.

Decontamination

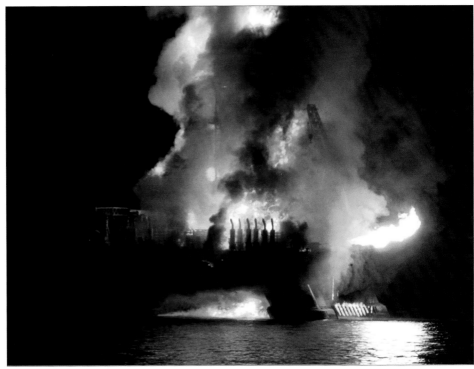

Fig. 9.1 Deepwater Horizon Explosion (2010), Courtesy of US Coast Guard

CASE SCENARIO

The Deepwater Horizon was a mobile offshore drilling unit located in the Gulf of Mexico. On April 20, 2010, a massive explosion occurred on the rig due to a wellhead blowout. Eleven workers were killed and seventeen injured. After burning for approximately 36 hours despite efforts to douse the flames, the Deepwater Horizon drilling unit sank. An oil leak from the blowout well was discovered on the same day when a large oil slick began to spread at the former rig site. On July 15, 2010 the leak was finally stopped by capping the gushing wellhead. An estimated 53,000 barrels of oil per day escaped from the well before it was capped, making the Deepwater Horizon oil spill the largest accidental marine oil spill in the history of the petroleum industry. The oil spill resulted in extensive contamination of the Gulf Coast.

Introduction

Decontamination is the removal of hazardous materials (biological, chemical or radioactive) from contaminated persons or equipment without further contaminating the casualty, environment or rescuers. The hazardous materials can be in the form of solids, liquids, or vapors.

Decontamination may be necessary following both natural and man-made disasters. Events such as the terrorist attack in Tokyo with the nerve agent Sarin have shown that up to 85% of victims arrive at a healthcare facility without prehospital treatment or decontamination. In terrorist attacks involving biological, chemical or radioactive agents, the "worried well" will also flood medical facilities, adding to the chaos and increasing the possibility that they too may become contaminated.

Decontamination has the following objectives:

- Prevention of further harm to the patient from the effects of the contaminating substances.

- Protection of the healthcare providers treating the patient from the hazardous agents.

- Ensuring that the hospital, and in particular the emergency department, does not become secondarily contaminated.

- Prevention of the spread of the contaminants to other persons and to the surrounding environment. The hospital must be able to recognize that an event has occurred and be prepared to handle the influx of patients arriving at the hospital.

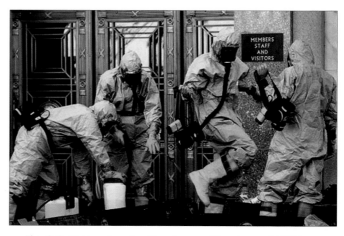

Fig. 9.2 Decontamination team, Courtesy of US Navy

Personal Protective Equipment

To safely perform decontamination, personnel must be in the appropriate level of personal protective equipment (PPE).

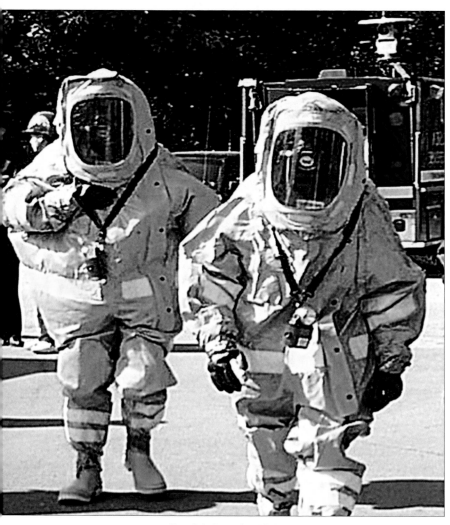

Fig. 9.3 Level A PPE

Level A PPE provides the highest level of skin, eye, and respiratory protection. It consists of a totally encapsulating, chemical-protective suit that is resistant to exposure by particulates, liquids, and vapors. It requires its own air supply, which is usually a positive-pressure self-contained breathing apparatus (SCBA), or other National Institute for Occupational Safety and Health (NIOSH) approved devices.

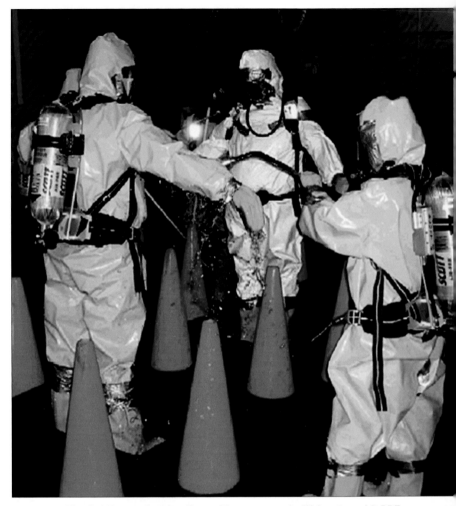

Fig. 9.4 Decontamination with personnel utilizing Level B PPE

Level B protection provides the same high level of respiratory and eye protection as Level A, but not as much skin protection. It consists of a positive pressure, self-contained breathing apparatus (SCBA) or other NIOSH approved devices. This is the usual level of protection that personnel will wear on the decontamination line.

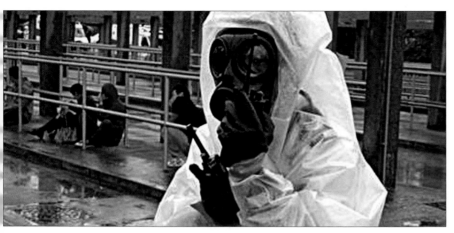

Fig. 9.5 Level C PPE

Level C PPE is usually worn when the substance and its concentration are known. The safety officer will determine when this level of protection is appropriate. Equipment consists of air-purifying respirators and chemically-resistant clothing.

Level D is minimal protection and consists of universal precautions equipment such as surgical gown, gloves, mask, and eye protection.

Types of Decontamination

The choice of decontamination technique will depend on:
* Number of casualties
* Severity of contamination
* Severity of injuries
* Available resources

Gross (Partial) Decontamination

Gross decontamination consists of removing the patient's clothing and jewelry, and, if possible, irrigating the patient's entire body with water. Casualties may be rinsed off with water hoses and sprays. This will remove about 85% of all contaminants from the patient. Gross decontamination should occur before the patient arrives at the hospital if at all possible.

Complete (Full) Decontamination

On-site decontamination is preferable, but is expensive and time-consuming. Portable decontamination tents are available to facilitate this process. On-site decontamination has the following advantages:
* Decreases contamination duration
* Decreases contamination of apparatus
* Decreases risk to hospital personnel

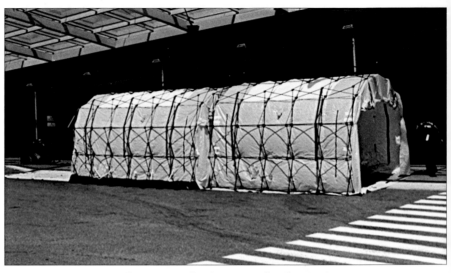

Fig. 9.6 Mobile decontamination tent

At the medical facility, the decontamination site should be separate from emergency room entrance to protect the facility and its personnel from being contaminated.

Decontamination Site

The site of decontamination is arranged in three zones: the Hot Zone, The Warm Zone, and the Cold Zone.

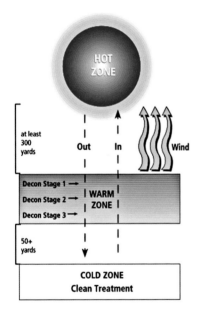

The **HOT ZONE** or the immediate isolation zone is the area of contamination. This area should be isolated immediately with access and egress controlled to avoid further contamination and casualties.

The **WARM ZONE** is located next to the Hot Zone. This is the zone where decontamination takes place. The Warm Zone should be established **"upwind"** from the Hot Zone. Low-lying areas where heavier-than-air vapors can settle and "run off" can accumulate should be avoided. The type and concentration of agent, meteorological conditions, dispersion and plume dynamics, and safe escape or evacuation routes must be considered in choosing this site. Personnel and patient safety are important priorities at all times.

The **COLD ZONE** is the area where the decontaminated patient is taken for definitive care if needed and disposition (transfer to other facilities or discharged). This area is adjacent to the Warm Zone, with the main patient area located 50 yards upwind from the Warm/Cold border. In this transition area, the patient is monitored for any lingering contamination that might have been missed. If no evidence of contamination exists, the Warm Zone decontamination team transfers the patient from the "dirty" side to the "clean" side.

82

Decontamination Techniques

Ambulatory patients should be instructed to peel off their clothes carefully from top to bottom to avoid aerosolizing any contaminates. They should then be instructed to wash themselves down with soap and water in the " head back" position to avoid contaminate running from the head into the eyes and mouth.

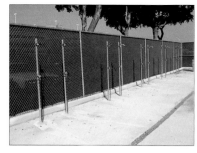

Fig. 9.7 Decontamination station for ambulatory patents

Non-ambulatory patients should have their clothes removed by personnel in the decontamination line. Clothes are removed starting at the midline and rolling the clothes to the sides of the patient, once again avoiding contamination of the newly exposed skin. Soap and water with a very soft brush are usually adequate to decontaminate the patient. A 0.5% hypochlorite solution (nine parts water or saline to 1 part bleach) followed by a copious water rinse is used mainly for equipment decontamination by civilian teams, but can be used as an agent for decontamination. This solution may also be used for irrigating open wounds (except open chest, abdominal, and cranial wounds). It can remove, oxidize, or hydrolyze most agents.

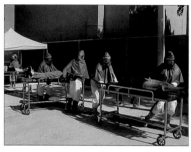

Fig. 9.8 Decontamination of non-ambulatory patients

Personnel should avoid abrading the skin when scrubbing the patient. This leads to open wounds that can introduce contaminate into the body.

- Eyes should be washed with copious amounts of Normal Saline.
- Fingernails should also be cleaned with a brush.
- Runoff from decontamination should be contained if possible to avoid contamination of the environment.
- A Redressing Station should be located at the end of the decontamination area near the Cold Zone and treatment area.

Full decontamination can be performed in PPE that is **one level below** what the Hot Zone entry team is wearing. The Safety Officer should make that determination whenever possible. Decontamination can take up to 20 minutes per casualty to perform complete decontamination. This should be taken into account when planning for a mass casualty event.

Triage may be performed in the Hot Zone by medical personnel in appropriate PPE. Casualties requiring medical treatment prior to going through decontamination are sent to a treatment area where medical issues can be addressed. Delivery of intramuscular (IM) antidotes and simple life-saving medical procedures, such as control of hemorrhage, can be administered to casualties awaiting decontamination by

FIELD OBSERVATION

The Triage Officer must possess critical knowledge of:

- **Natural course of injuries**
- **Available medical resources**
- **Medical evacuation capacity**

medical personnel wearing appropriate protective gear. The patient can then be sent to undergo decontamination or evacuated to a facility that is a higher level of care.

Special Considerations
Biological
Soap and water are adequate to decontaminate these types of patients. A respirator (TB equivalent) or a N95 mask with Tyvek suit, gloves, and eye protection is adequate PPE for rescuers.

Chemical
Time is of the essence in many chemical exposures. Decontamination should start as quickly as possible to decrease contact time with the agent. There are many agent-specific detectors available that can be used to monitor how effectively decontamination has been performed. They should be used to monitor casualties who have undergone decontamination.

Radioactive
Time, distance, and shielding are important factors to reduce exposure to the rescuer. The greater the time spent in the environment, the greater the dose of radiation. Similarly, a large quantity of radiation in the environment leads to more exposure and a higher dose of radiation. Doubling the distance from the source of radiation will decrease the exposure by a factor of four. Therefore, when decontaminating a casualty, long-handled brushes should be used to gently scrub the victim. Swabs from the ears, nose, and mouth should be obtained for monitoring purposes.

Internal decontamination using enteral absorption blockade (e.g., Prussian blue), end-organ uptake blockade (e.g., potassium iodide) or chelation (e.g., pentetate calcium trisodium [Ca-DTPA]) should be considered in those casualties exposed to specific types of isotopes. Prussian blue can increase the elimination of cesium and thallium. Potassium Iodide can block radioactive iodine uptake into the thyroid gland. Pentetate calcium trisodium can bind americium, curium, and plutonium, enhancing their renal elimination.

Decontamination Drills

Decontamination drills are an essential part of disaster preparedness. Practical drills will enhance efficiency and confidence in decontamination.

RISK ALERT!

The cardinal rule for protection against radioactive substances is TIME, DISTANCE, and SHIELDING.

The actual composition of the decontamination team will vary, but, in general, include the following personnel:

- Team leader
- Triage officer
- Medical personnel
- Decontamination personnel
- Transport personnel
- Security personnel

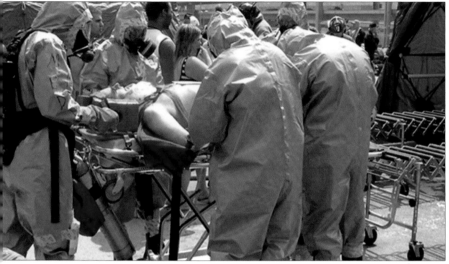
Fig. 9.9 Decontamination drill

Summary

The basic principles in response to ANY hazardous-material incident are the same regardless of the agents involved. Removal of the outer layers of clothing may reduce contamination by up to 85%. It is important for medical providers to protect themselves during decontamination with the appropriate level of PPE.

KEY POINTS

In a mass casualty incident, removal of the patient's clothing and jewelry will reduce contamination by approximately 85%.

Medical responders must utilize the appropriate PPE when triaging and decontaminating "contaminated" victims.

Triage category for decontamination may be different from the triage category for medical treatment. (For example, a liquid nerve agent casualty may be stable medically, but needs immediate decontamination.)

Biological Agents

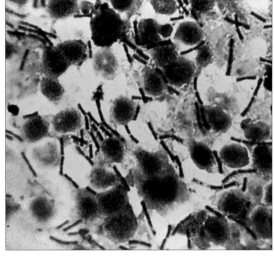

Fig.10.1 Bacillus anthracis, Courtesy of CDC

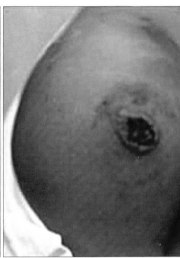

Fig.10.2 Cutaneous anthrax,
Courtesy of CDC

CASE SCENARIO

The 2001 anthrax attacks in the United States occurred over the course of several weeks beginning on September 18, 2001. At least 22 people developed anthrax infections, with 11 life-threatening inhalational anthrax infections. Five individuals died of inhalational anthrax. The type of anthrax was identified as the Ames strain of the bacterium.

Introduction

Exposure to biological agents may be accidental or intentional. **Biological terrorism is the intentional use of microorganisms or toxins derived from living organisms to kill or injure humans, animals, or plants.** Some biological agents can serve dual purposes. Botulinum toxin, for example, has several therapeutic uses, including the treatment of certain neuromuscular disorders as well as cosmetic use in medicine.

Past events, including the anthrax mail attacks of 2001, have demonstrated the vulnerability of civilian populations to the threat of biological agents. The following organisms and toxins are believed to have the greatest potential for use as bioterrorism weapons:

- Bacillus anthracis (Anthrax) - Bacteria
- Yersinia pestis (Plague) – Bacteria
- Francisella tularensis (Tularemia) - Bacteria
- Botulinum toxins (Botulism) - Toxins
- Variola major (Smallpox) - Virus
- Hemorrhagic fever viruses such as Ebola and Marburg

The above six are known as "Category A" bioterrorism agents (CDC classification). Other agents that also have potential as bioterrorism threats include encephalitis viruses such as VEE (Venezuelan Equine Encephalitis), toxins such as Ricin, Staphylococcal Enterotoxin B (SEB), and the trichothecene mycotoxins, and bacteria such as the causative agents of Glanders and Melioidosis (*Burkholderia* species), Brucellosis (Brucella species), Q Fever (*Coxiella burnetii*), and Typhus (*Rickettsia prowazekii*).

Routes of Exposure

Inhalation

The route of exposure of most concern with biological agents, especially terrorist attacks, is inhalation of the agent. In an attack, a terrorist might attempt to generate aerosols of the biological agent composed of particles of the right size and diameter to be inhaled deeply into the lungs, where they could begin to cause illness. The aerosol would be odorless, colorless, and invisible due to its small particle size. Inhalation was the route of exposure that caused five deaths during the anthrax mail attacks in the United States in 2001.

Oral

The oral route for biological agents is believed to be less important, but is still significant. Contamination of food may occur directly or secondarily after an aerosol attack and may represent a hazard for infection or intoxication by ingestion. Ensuring an uncontaminated food and water supply is an important function of public health, and should be a priority after a biological attack.

Dermal

Intact skin provides the most effective barrier for many, but not all, biological agents. Some bacteria, viruses, and toxins can penetrate mucous membranes and abraded or otherwise damaged skin, so these should be protected in the event of an attack.

FIELD OBSERVATION:
Indications of Possible Biological Attack

- A disease entity that is unusual or that does not occur naturally in a given geographic area, or combinations of unusual disease entities in the same patient populations

- Multiple disease entities in the same patients, indicating that mixed agents may have been used in the attack

- Large numbers of both military and civilian casualties when such populations inhabit the same area

- Data suggesting a massive point-source or line-source outbreak (for non-contagious agents)

- Apparent aerosol route of infection

- High morbidity and mortality relative to the number of personnel at risk

- Illness limited to fairly localized or circumscribed geographical areas or workplaces

- Low attack rates in personnel who work in areas with filtered air supplies or closed ventilation systems

- Sentinel dead animals of multiple species

Responding to a Biological Attack

Physical Protection

The most effective and important protection against biological agents is physical protection. A full-face respirator prevents exposure of the respiratory tract and mucous membranes, including conjunctivae, to infectious or toxic agents, theoretically obviating the need for additional measures. However, given the imperfect state of detection technology today, these measures may be impractical, especially in civilian populations.

Decontamination

Any dermal exposure should be treated immediately by washing with soap and water. In addition, medical responders must guard against secondary contamination (i.e., contamination passed from the clothing of affected individuals) through the use of appropriate physical protection until decontamination is complete.

- Toxin-exposed victims can be dealt with routinely, and patients affected by botulinum toxin or staphylococcal enterotoxin B (SEB) present no risk to providers (except through contaminated clothing).

- Anthrax could present a risk from open skin lesions or blood of victims, potentially causing cutaneous anthrax in medical responders. Once decontaminated, universal or standard precautions should be adequate to protect those treating anthrax casualties.

- Postmortem examinations of suspected anthrax victims should be performed with strict mask, gown, and glove precautions because of the large numbers of organisms in body fluids. If procedures that generate blood aerosols are conducted, measures should be taken to protect the respiratory tract.

Prophylaxis and Therapy

Medical defenses against some biological agents are limited. High-dose agent exposure near the sources of dissemination may possibly overwhelm any medical protective measures. While the precise efficacy of available medical countermeasures has never been evaluated in actual field circumstances, it can be inferred from laboratory studies on nonhuman primates. While these extrapolations may not be exact, they strongly support the efficacy of vaccines and drugs for individuals exposed to high levels of some agents. At some point in the future, it may become appropriate for certain key civilian personnel to be immunized against major threat agents, such as anthrax and smallpox.

Response to Bacterial Agents

Anthrax *(Bacillus anthracis)*

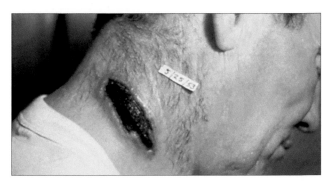

Fig. 10.3 Cutaneous anthrax lesion, Courtesy of CDC

An aerosolized attack with anthrax spores would cause inhalational anthrax, a rare form of the naturally occurring disease. The incubation period is generally 1-6 days, although longer periods have been noted.

Clinical Effects

- Fever, malaise, fatigue, cough, and mild chest discomfort are the first clinical symptoms.

- Disease progresses in 2-3 days to severe respiratory distress with dyspnea, diaphoresis, stridor, cyanosis, and shock.

- Death typically occurs within 24-36 hours after onset of severe symptoms.

Physical findings may include evidence of pleural effusions and meningitis, both of which may be hemorrhagic, and edema of the chest wall.

Prophylaxis

A vaccine for anthrax (Anthrax Vaccine Absorbed - AVA) is available. It is an FDA-approved, protective antigen (PA)-based, non-live vaccine that contains no anthrax organisms. It is given in a 5-dose series (IM) at 0 and 4 weeks and 6, 12, and 18 months (primary series with yearly boosters, if needed). In non-human primate studies, this vaccine has protected animals against over 500 lethal doses (LD50s) of anthrax spores.

The antibiotics ciprofloxacin and doxycycline also provide prophylaxis against anthrax. In the event of attack, one of these drugs should be administered to exposed individuals and continued for at least 8 weeks if the vaccine is not available and for at least 4 weeks in combination with the vaccine.

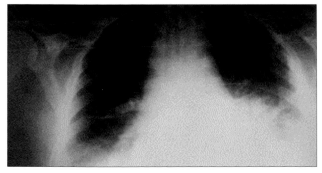

*Fig. 10.4 Widened mediastinum characteristic
of inhalational anthrax, Courtesy of CDC*

**INHALATIONAL
ANTHRAX TREATMENT**

- Treat at earliest
  sign of disease
- Ciprofloxacin 400
  mg IV q 12 hours
  OR
- Doxycycline 200
  mg IV, followed by
  doxycycline 100
  mg IV q 12 hours

Treatment

The case fatality rate for the rare cases of inhalational anthrax has been 80-90% historically. However, in the 2001 mail anthrax attacks in the United States, six of eleven inhalational anthrax casualties were saved with modern intensive care and treatment.

Most naturally occurring strains of anthrax are sensitive to penicillin. However, IV ciprofloxacin and doxycycline are the treatments of choice for inhalational anthrax. Potential alternative treatments include gentamicin, erythromycin, and chloramphenicol. In addition, intensive supportive therapy for shock, fluid volume deficit, and maintenance of respiration may all be needed.

Plague *(Yersinia pestis)*

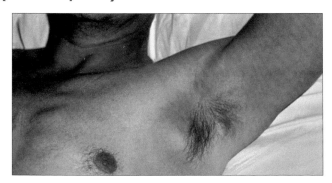

*Fig. 10.5 Swollen lymph glands (buboes) often occur
in the neck, armpit, and inguinal regions of bubonic
plague victims, Courtesy of CDC*

Under natural conditions, humans are infected by this bacterial disease primarily through the bites of rodents' fleas. The disease takes three clinical forms: bubonic, primary septicemic, and pneumonic.

In a biological attack, the plague bacillus would most likely be disseminated by aerosol, producing the pneumonic form of the disease.

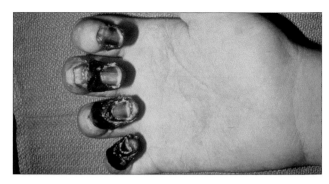

Fig.10.6 Gangrene of the digits due to plague, Courtesy of CDC

PLAGUE TREATMENT

- Streptomycin 30 mg/kg/day IM in 2 divided doses,

  OR

- Gentamicin 5 mg/kg IV once daily

  OR

- Ciprofloxacin 400 mg IV q 12 hours

Clinical Effects

Bubonic Plague

Bubonic plague, featuring high fever, malaise and swollen, painful lymph nodes may progress spontaneously to the septicemic form (shock, thrombosis, disseminated intravascular coagulation or DIC), or to the pneumonic form. There is a 50% case-fatality rate in untreated patients because of circulatory collapse, bleeding diathesis, and peripheral thrombosis.

Pneumonic Plague

The incubation period for pneumonic plague is 2-3 days, and onset is acute and fulminant with malaise, high fever, chills, headache, myalgia, cough with bloody sputum, and toxemia. Pneumonia progresses rapidly, resulting in respiratory insufficiency manifesting as dyspnea and cyanosis. There is close to 100% mortality in untreated patients due to respiratory failure, circulatory collapse, and bleeding diathesis.

Prophylaxis

For asymptomatic persons exposed to either a plague aerosol or to a patient with suspected pneumonic plague, give doxycycline 100 mg orally twice daily for 7 days, or the duration of risk of exposure plus 1 week. Alternative antibiotics include ciprofloxacin, tetracycline, or chloramphenicol.

Treatment

Streptomycin, gentamicin, doxycycline, or ciprofloxacin are effective if begun early for pneumonic plague. Treatment should be initiated within 24 hours of onset of symptoms.

However, since streptomycin may not be available today, gentamicin may be the most readily available antibiotic for treatment of a patient infected with *Yersinia pestis*.

Supportive management of life-threatening complications, such as shock, hyperpyrexia (high fever), convulsions, and DIC must be initiated when these complications arise.

Tularemia *(Francisella tularensis)*

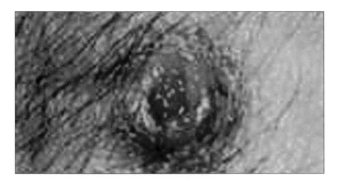

Fig.10.7 Tularemia, Courtesy of CDC

Clinical Effects

Under natural conditions, humans contract this bacterial disease through inoculation of skin or mucous membranes with blood or tissue fluids of infected animals, or bites of infected deerflies, mosquitoes, or ticks. Three major clinical forms are generally seen, although there are six different clinical syndromes associated with tularemia.

- *Ulceroglandular* tularemia generally presents with a local ulcer and regional lymphadenopathy, fever, chills, headache, and malaise.

- *Typhoidal* (septicemic) tularemia presents with fever, headache, malaise, prostration, and weight loss. A significant pneumonia may exist as well, with substernal discomfort and a non-productive cough.

- *Pneumonic* tularemia is a severe atypical pneumonia that may be fulminant and is associated with a high case-fatality rate if untreated. It can be primary following inhalation of organisms or secondary following hematogenous/septicemic spread. It is seen in 30–80% of the typhoidal cases and in 10–15% of the ulceroglandular cases. **This is the form of the disease that will be most likely seen following an aerosol biological attack.** One factor that makes tularemia an unusually dangerous biological threat agent when dispensed by aerosol is its very low infectious dose – as low as ten to fifty organisms.

Prophylaxis

A vaccine (live vaccine strain or LVS) may be available as an investigational new drug. It is administered once by scarification. A 2-week course of antibiotics is generally effective as prophylaxis when given after exposure.

Treatment

Streptomycin has historically been the treatment of choice for tularemia; however, it may not be readily available immediately after a large-scale biological attack. Therefore, gentamicin and other alternative drugs should be considered as first-line treatments.

TULAREMIA PROPHYLAXIS

- Ciprofloxacin 500 mg po bid for 2 weeks

  OR

- Doxycycline 100 mg po bid for 2 weeks

  OR

- Tetracycline 500 mg po q 6 hours for 2 weeks

TULAREMIA TREATMENT

- Streptomycin 7.5–10 mg/kg IM q 12 hours for 10-14 days

  OR

- Gentamicin 3-5 mg/kg/day IV for 10-14 days

  OR

- Ciprofloxacin 750 mg po q 12 hours for 10-14 days

Response to Viral Agents

Smallpox *(Variola)*

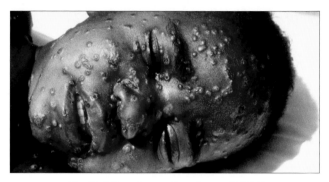

Fig.10.8 Smallpox, Courtesy of CDC

SMALLPOX LESIONS

- All same stage of development
- Painful
- Deep skin lesions
- More abundant on extremities and face (centrifugal distribution)

CHICKENPOX LESIONS

- Multiple stages of development
- Pruritic
- Superficial lesions
- Centripetal (central) distribution

Smallpox is a disease caused by an Orthopox virus, *Variola*. Despite the global eradication of smallpox and continued availability of a vaccine, potential weaponization of *Variola* continues to pose a terrorist threat because of its aerosol infectivity, the relative ease of large-scale production, and a population that is no longer immune to the virus.

Vaccination programs in the United States were stopped during the late 1970s and early 1980s. Most adults in the United States have not been immunized in at least 20 years, and most young people under age 32 have no smallpox immunity. One case of smallpox would be considered a public health emergency of the highest order.

Clinical Effects

- The incubation period of smallpox averages 12 days and ranges from 7-19 days following exposure.

- Clinical manifestations begin acutely with malaise, fever, rigors, vomiting, headache, and backache. 15% of patients develop delirium.

- Following eruptions on the face and upper and lower extremities (centrifugal distribution as opposed to varicella, which has a centripetal [central] distribution initially), the rash spreads centrally to the trunk over the next week. Lesions quickly progress from macules to papules and eventually to pustular vesicles, all generally at the same rate of development. This is in contrast with varicella where lesions may be present simultaneously in different stages of development.

- Clinically, smallpox is difficult to distinguish from varicella (chickenpox), monkeypox, or cowpox.

Prophylaxis

Immediate vaccination or revaccination should be undertaken for all exposed individuals. In the civilian setting, strict quarantine of asymptomatic contacts may prove to be impractical and impossible to enforce. A reasonable alternative would be to require contacts to stay at home and check their temperatures daily. Any fever above 38°C (101°F) during the 17-day period following exposure to a confirmed case would suggest the possible development of smallpox. The contact should then be isolated immediately, preferably at home, until smallpox is either confirmed or ruled out and remain in isolation until all scabs separate.

Treatment

At present, there is no licensed effective therapy for smallpox, and treatment of a clinical case remains supportive. Vaccinia vaccination and possibly vaccinia immune globulin possess some efficacy in post-exposure prophylaxis.

Antivirals for use against smallpox are under investigation. Cidofovir and its analogs have been shown to have significant in vitro and in vivo activity in experimental animals – however, it has significant potential adverse side effects. Other experimental compounds and monoclonal antibodies are under development. Further studies of these therapies are ongoing.

Isolation and Decontamination

Smallpox is extremely contagious. **Droplet and airborne precautions must be maintained for a minimum of 17 days following exposure for all contacts.** Patients should be considered infectious until all scabs separate and should be quarantined during this period.

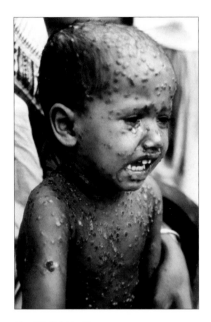

Fig.10.9 Smallpox, Courtesy of CDC

Venezuelan Equine Encephalitis (VEE)

Venezuelan equine encephalitis (VEE) is a viral infection that can cause severe disease in humans as well as in Equidae (horses, mules, burros, and donkeys). Natural infections are acquired by the bites of a wide variety of mosquitoes. Equidae serve as amplifying hosts and the source of mosquito infection.

Clinical Effects

VEE treatment is supportive only. Treat uncomplicated VEE infections with analgesics to relieve headache and myalgia.

- The incubation period is 1-6 days. The onset is sudden with generalized malaise, spiking fevers, rigors, severe headache, photophobia, and myalgias in the legs and lumbosacral area.

- Nausea, vomiting, cough, sore throat, and diarrhea may follow.

The clinical syndrome is similar to influenza, and the acute phase lasts 24-72 hours and is sometimes followed by a long period of asthenia and lethargy with full health regained only after 1–2 weeks. **The incidence of CNS disease and associated morbidity and mortality would be much higher after a bioterrorist attack, especially in children.** The treatment of VEE is supportive only.

Prophylaxis

A live, attenuated IND vaccine (TC-83) exists, which is given as a single subcutaneous 0.5 mg dose. Febrile reactions occur in 18% of persons vaccinated, and approximately 10% fail to develop detectable neutralizing antibodies. A second formalin-inactivated, killed vaccine (C-84) is used to boost antibody titers in those receiving the live vaccine.

In animal experiments, antiretroviral drugs, including interferon-alpha, have proven effective for post-exposure prophylaxis of VEE. There are no clinical data in humans.

Treatment

No specific antiviral therapy exists; hence, treatment is supportive only. Patients with uncomplicated VEE infection may be treated with analgesics to relieve headache and myalgia. Patients who develop encephalitis may require anticonvulsants and intensive supportive care to maintain fluid and electrolyte balance, ensure adequate ventilation, and avoid complicating secondary bacterial infections.

Patients should be treated in a screened room or in quarters treated with a residual insecticide for at least 5 days after onset, or until afebrile. Human cases may be infectious (via mosquito vector) for at least 72 hours due to viremia.

Response to Biological Toxins

Botulinum Toxins

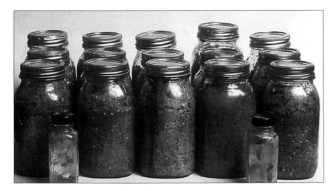

Fig. 10.10 Food (jalapeno peppers) contaminated with botulinum, Courtesy of CDC

Clinical Effects

- **Symptoms usually begin with cranial nerve palsies**, including ptosis (drooping of the upper eyelids), blurred vision, diplopia (double vision), dry mouth and throat, dysphagia (difficulty swallowing), and dysphonia (difficulty speaking).

- This is followed by symmetrical descending flaccid paralysis, with generalized weakness and progression to respiratory failure.

- Symptoms begin as early as 12–36 hours after inhalation, but may take several days after exposure to low doses of toxin.

Prophylaxis

A pentavalent vaccine exists as an IND product and is used in the laboratory setting for those working with botulinum toxins. This vaccine has potency issues and may not be effective against some neurotoxin serotypes. The Department of Defense is developing a new recombinant botulinum vaccine that will be effective against botulinum toxin types A and B.

Treatment

- Early administration of heptavalent antitoxin (IND product) may prevent or slow progression to respiratory failure. There is now a significant amount of recently produced IND despeciated heptavalent equine-derived antitoxin available from the US Strategic National (pharmaceutical) Stockpile (SNS), administered by CDC.

- Intubation and ventilatory assistance for respiratory failure. Tracheostomy may be required.

FIELD OBSERVATION

The occurrence of an epidemic of afebrile patients with progressive symmetrical descending flaccid paralysis strongly suggests botulinum intoxication.

BOTULINUM TOXIN TREATMENT

- Early administration of trivalent or heptavalent antitoxin, if available

- Intubation for ventilatory assistance

Staphylococcal Enterotoxin B (SEB)

Clinical Effects

- A latent period of 3-12 hours after aerosol exposure is followed by sudden onset of fever, chills, headache, myalgia, and non-productive cough. Some patients may develop shortness of breath and retrosternal chest pain.

- Patients tend to plateau rapidly to a fairly stable clinical state. Fever may last 2-5 days, and cough may persist for up to 4 weeks. Patients may also present with nausea, vomiting, and diarrhea if they swallow the toxin.

- Severe cases may manifest acute pulmonary edema and respiratory failure.

Prophylaxis

There is no licensed vaccine available.

Treatment

Treatment is limited to supportive care. Artificial ventilation might be needed for very severe cases, and attention to fluid management is important.

T-2 Mycotoxins

Clinical Effects

- Exposure to these fungus-produced toxins causes skin pain, pruritus, redness, vesicles, necrosis, and sloughing of the epidermis.

- Airway effects include nose and throat pain, rhinorrhea, itching and sneezing, cough, dyspnea, wheezing, chest pain, and *hemoptysis* (coughing up blood). The toxins may also produce adverse effects after ingestion or eye contact.

- Severe intoxication from exposure to a large amount of toxin may result in prostration, weakness, ataxia, collapse, shock, and death.

Prophylaxis

There is no vaccine available.

Treatment

There is no specific antidote. Treatment is supportive. Soap and water washing, even 4-6 hours after exposure, can significantly reduce dermal toxicity. Washing within 1 hour may prevent toxicity entirely. Super-activated charcoal should be given orally if the toxin is swallowed.

SEB TREATMENT

Supportive measures, including ventilatory assistance as needed.

FIELD OBSERVATION

T-2 Mycotoxins should be suspected if an aerosol attack occurs in the form of "yellow rain" with droplets of variously pigmented oily fluids contaminating clothes and the environment.

Ricin

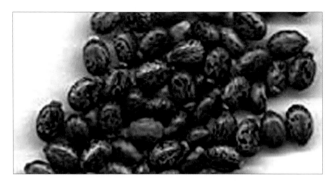

Fig. 10.11 Castor beans, source of Ricin, Courtesy of CDC

Clinical Effects

- When inhaled, this toxin may produce pathologic changes within 8 hours and severe respiratory symptoms followed by acute respiratory failure.

- When ingested, ricin causes severe gastrointestinal symptoms followed by vascular collapse and death.

- Acute onset of fever, chest tightness, cough, dyspnea, nausea, and arthralgias occurs 4–8 hours after inhalational exposure.

- Airway necrosis and pulmonary capillary leak resulting in pulmonary edema would likely occur within 18–24 hours and death in 36–72 hours.

Prophylaxis

There is currently no vaccine or prophylactic antitoxin available for human use.

Treatment

Management is supportive and should include treatment for pulmonary edema. Gastric lavage and cathartics are indicated for ingestion, but charcoal is of little value for large molecules such as Ricin.

FIELD OBSERVATION

Acute lung injury in large numbers of geographically clustered patients suggests exposure to aerosolized ricin.

The rapid time course to severe symptoms and death is unusual for infectious agents and should also suggest ricin.

RICIN TREATMENT

- Thorough decontamination of skin with soap and water, and flush eyes with water or Normal Saline if exposed

- Supportive treatment for pulmonary edema

- Gastric lavage for ingestion

Characteristics of Selected Biological Agents

Disease	Transmit Person to Person?	Incubation Period	Duration of Illness	Case-Fatality Rate	Persistence of Organism in Environment	Vaccine Efficacy (aerosol exposure)
Inhalational anthrax	No	1-6 days	3-5 days (usually fatal if untreated)	High	Very stable – spores remain viable in soil for > 40 years	Tested effective in primates
Cholera	Rare	4 hrs - 5 days usually (2-3 days)	>1 week	Low with treatment; High without treatment	Unstable in aerosols & fresh water; stable in salt water	No data on aerosol
Pneumonic Plague	High with close contact	2-3 days	1-6 days (usually fatal)	High unless treated within 12-24 hrs	For up to 1 year in soil; 270 days in live tissue	Vaccine no longer available – did not protect against aerosol exposure
Tularemia	No	2-10 days (avg. 3-5)	>2 weeks	Moderate if untreated	For months in moist soil or other media	80% protection in animals
Smallpox	High	7-17 days (avg. 12)	Up to 4 weeks	High to moderate	Very stable	Vaccine protective in primates
Venezuelan Equine Encephalitis	Low	2-6 days	Days to weeks	Low	Relatively unstable	Vaccine protective in hamsters
Viral Hemorrhagic Fevers	Moderate	4-21 days	Death between 7-16 days	Moderate (High for Zaire strain)	Relatively unstable– depends on agent	No vaccines
Botulism	No	1-5 days	Death in 24-72 hours; lasts months if not lethal	High without respiratory support	For weeks in non-moving water or food	3-dose efficacy 100% in primates
Staph Enterotoxin B	No	3-12 hours after inhalation	Hours	<1%	Resistant to freezing	No vaccine
Ricin	No	18-24 hours	Days–death within 10-12 days for ingestion	High	Stable	No vaccine

Summary

Individuals may be exposed to biological agents either accidentally or as a result of biological terrorism. The route of exposure of most concern is inhalation of the biological agent. Medical defenses against some of the agents are limited. The most effective and most important protection against biological agents is physical protection.

KEY POINTS

 Biological agents most likely to be used as weapons of terrorism include anthrax, smallpox, plague, tularemia, botulinum toxins, and hemorrhagic fever viruses such as Ebola and Marburg.

 Vaccines are available to protect against some biological agents (anthrax, smallpox), and antibiotics may be effective against bacterial agents such as anthrax, plague, and tularemia, if given early enough.

 Antitoxins may slow or stop progression of clinical botulism if given early in the course of illness.

Chemical Agents

Chapter 11

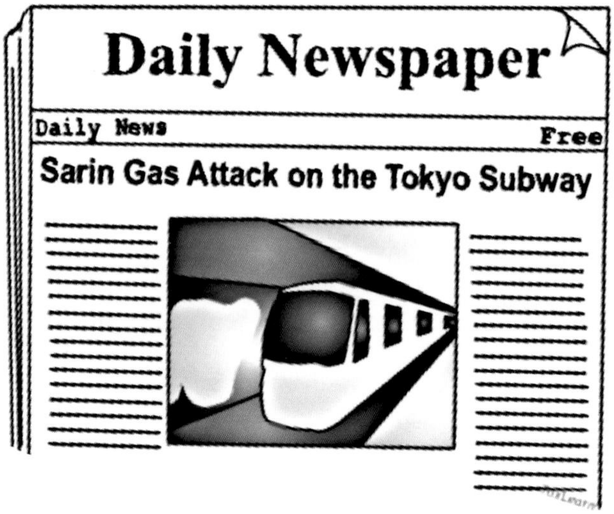

Fig.11.1 Sarin attack, Tokyo (1995), Courtesy of National Library of Medicine

CASE SCENARIO

On March 20, 1995, terrorism changed when terrorists used a chemical agent against a civilian population. The nerve agent sarin (GB) was released in the Tokyo subway system by the terrorist group, the Aum Shinrikyo cult, resulting in exposure of victims, rescuers, and hospital staff. In addition to the victims experiencing physical effects of the sarin gas, many presented with psychological effects. One hundred-thirty-five (135) of 1,364 emergency medical personnel involved in victim rescue were contaminated. Twenty-three percent (23%) of medical staff in area hospitals were contaminated.

The Editor and Author would like to acknowledge the valuable contribution of Frederick R. Sidell MD (Deceased) to the Chemical Agent Chapter. Dr. Sidell was an internationally-recognized expert on chemical agents. We are grateful for his commitment to this educational project.

Introduction

Release of chemical agents may be unintentional (industrial accidents) or intentional (terrorism). Most chemical warfare agents are liquids that must be dispersed to be maximally effective. This can be done in three general ways:

- Aerosolizing the liquid with a sprayer (such as is done with pesticides)
- Aerosolizing the liquid with an explosion
- Allowing the liquid to evaporate and dispersing the resulting vapor

When used outside, a vapor generally will not remain in place because even a light wind will dilute and carry it away. However, when dispersed inside a structure where no wind is present, a vapor can remain and its concentration will increase until the ventilation system removes it from inside, dispersing it even farther outside the structure.

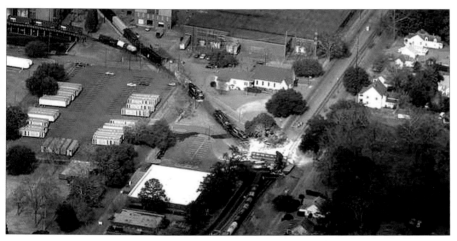

Fig. 11.2 Train crash involving tankers containing chlorine gas, Graniteville, South Carolina (2005), Courtesy of Environmental Protection Agency

There are six classes of chemical agents that are discussed in this chapter:

- Nerve agents
- Vesicants (blistering agents)
- Hydrogen cyanide
- Pulmonary agents
- Incapacitating agents
- Riot control agents

Characteristics of Chemical Agents

Most agents listed here are liquids, with the exception of some riot control agents, which are solids, and phosgene (boiling point = 8.2°C) and chlorine (boiling point = -34°C) that are gases at ambient temperatures. Liquid agents evaporate and produce a vapor hazard—some more than others. **The higher the vapor pressure, the more volatile the substance, and the more likely it is to evaporate, causing a vapor hazard.**

- Hydrogen cyanide (boiling point = 25.5°C; vapor pressure = 742 mm Hg at 25°C) is the **most volatile** liquid chemical agent at ambient temperature; e.g., most likely to evaporate and produce the greatest vapor hazard.

- Sulfur mustard (vapor pressure = 0.11 mm Hg at 25°C) and VX (vapor pressure = 0.0007 mm Hg at 25°C) are the **least volatile chemical agents**.

- These liquid agents, except hydrogen cyanide (specific gravity = 0.687), are heavier than water and can be covered by water when decontaminating terrain and objects.

- The vapor form of these agents, except hydrogen cyanide (vapor density = 0.94), is heavier than air (vapor density >1) and will sink into ditches, trenches, and basements. **Individuals are generally safer standing up than lying down in the presence of a chemical agent.**

- The direction and speed of the wind is a key factor as well. Individuals should try to remain upwind of a source.

- **Persistency is a key attribute of chemical agents and refers to the length of time a chemical agent will remain on objects or alternatively, how quickly the agent evaporates.** Persistency depends on the ambient temperature and the physical and chemical characteristics of the agent. If a chemical remains on the ground under temperate conditions without evaporating, it is considered to be persistent, such as VX.

Responding to a Chemical Attack

When responding to a chemical incident, one of the first things medical responders should do is establish a clean treatment area. This should be upwind of the contaminated area (the "hot zone") and at least 50 yards from the outer perimeter of the "warm zone." The inner perimeter of the "warm zone" should be at least 300 yards upwind from the source of contamination. Perimeters are best determined by consulting a software program that uses a plume modeling program, e. g., CAMEO or ALOHA. Medical responders must leave the hot zone only via a specially designated pathway, called an access corridor, into the warm zone where they will be decontaminated.

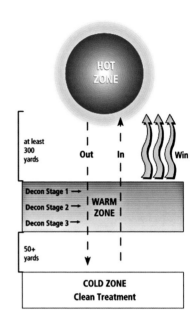

If there are multiple casualties who have severe, life-threatening injuries, two medical care responders should work in the contaminated area, one to triage and one to administer emergency care, including the administration of intramuscular nerve agent antidotes, intubation or ventilation with a bag-valve mask, and emergency first aid. These responders must be in full protective equipment, including mask, gloves, suit, etc. Even potentially life-saving emergency treatments in contaminated areas are limited by the practicalities of providing emergency care and administering medicines while in protective gear.

Nerve Agents

Nerve agents are very toxic relatives of organophosphate insecticides. They cause biological effects by disrupting the normal mechanisms by which nerves communicate with muscles, glands, and other nerves. This causes hyperactivity in these structures before they fatigue and stop functioning.

The important nerve agents are:

- GA (Tabun)
- GB (Sarin)
- GD (Soman)
- GF
- VX

Nerve agents enter the body either percutaneously (through the skin) or by inhalation (through the lungs).

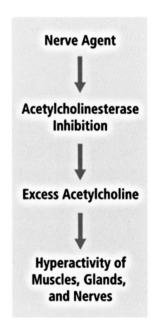

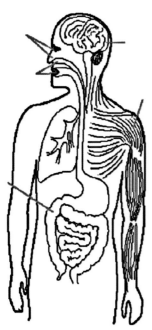

Fig.11.3 Cholinergic nervous system

All nerve agents inhibit the enzyme *acetylcholinesterase*. When inhibited, this enzyme cannot perform its normal function—breakdown (inactivation) of *acetylcholine*, the neurotransmitter in the cholinergic nervous system. **Acetylcholine then accumulates and over-stimulates muscles, glands, and other nerves.**

The cholinergic nervous system is divided into two sub-systems:

* Muscarinic
* Nicotinic

While nerve agents affect both of these sub-systems, their clinical presentations are different, and atropine works only on muscarinic receptors.

Clinical Effects

The clinical effects of nerve agents, summarized in the following chart, depend on:

* The route of exposure
* The amount of exposure to the agent (concentration of agent) and the exposure time
* Preexisting medical conditions, especially cardiac, pulmonary, or neuromuscular

Treatment

* Protect yourselves from exposure.
* Move casualties into the access corridor of the warm zone for decontamination as quickly as possible.
* Administer antidotes as soon as possible.
  o Atropine (IM in severe cases) is mainly to reverse bronchoconstriction and excessive secretions, and generally does not affect pupil size.
  o Pralidoxime (e.g., Pralidoxime chloride, 2-PAM, 2-PAMCl)
  o Diazepam for convulsions
* Ventilate casualties who are apneic as soon as possible.
  o Use bag-valve mask.
  o If ventilation is difficult, administer atropine IM to reduce resistance caused by bronchoconstriction.
  o Suction secretions as needed.

TREATMENT ALERT!

Nerve agent antidotes, atropine and Pralidoxime, can be given IM and should be administered as soon as practically possible.

106

Summary of Nerve Agent Effects and Treatment

VAPOR EXPOSURE:	Clinical Effects	Treatment
Mild	Unilateral or bilateral miosis (pinpoint pupils)	No treatment
	Rhinorrhea (runny nose)	2 mg atropine if rhinorrhea or discomfort is great
Moderate	Shortness of breath	2-4 mg atropine depending upon severity; repeat 2 mg doses every 5 minutes until improvement
		Ventilate as needed via bag-valve mask
Severe	Casualty is gasping for air, unconscious, or convulsing	6 mg atropine IM; repeat 2 mg doses every 5 minutes until improvement
		Pralidoxime (2-PAM) 1 g IV or 1.8 g IM
		Diazepam 10 mg autoinjector IM if convulsing
		Ventilate via bag-valve mask
		Suction airways if secretions are copious
LIQUID EXPOSURE:	**Clinical Effects**	**Treatment**
Mild	Localized sweating, fasciculations	2 mg atropine
		Pralidoxime (2-PAM) 1 g IV or 600 mg IM
Moderate	Gastrointestinal effects	2 mg atropine
		Pralidoxime (2-PAM) 1 g IV or 600 mg IM
Severe	Same as for vapor	Same as for vapor

Nerve Agent Antidotes

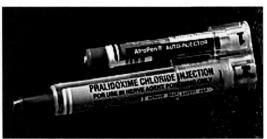

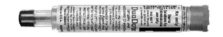

Fig.11.4 MARK 1 KIT – Atropine (2mg) and Pralidoxime Chloride Auto Injectors, Courtesy of CDC

Fig. 11.5 DuoDote – Auto Injector, Atropine and Pralidoxime, Courtesy of Meridian Medical Technologies

Vesicants

Vesicants are substances that cause *erythema* (redness) and *vesicles* (blisters) on the skin as well as injury to the eyes, the airways, and other organs. There are two vesicants considered in this chapter: sulfur mustard and Lewisite.

Sulfur Mustard

Sulfur mustard, a persistent agent, is an oily liquid, ranging in color from yellow to brown, depending upon the type and amount of impurities. Sulfur mustard enters the cells of the skin or mucous membranes and produces biochemical damage within seconds to minutes after contact with the vapor or liquid. Despite this rapid activity, clinical effects do not occur until hours later. **Contact with mustard does NOT cause immediate pain, redness, or other noticeable effects.**

Clinical Effects

Clinical effects of mustard exposure do not occur for hours after contact. Because of this, persons exposed to mustard do not need immediate medical care with the exception of decontamination as soon as possible. However, anyone suspected of being exposed to mustard should be <u>observed</u> for at least 8 hours after decontamination.

Eventually, mustard will cause:

- Red and blistering skin
- Irritation and other damage to the eyes, including possible scarring
- Damage to the lining of the airways, which, if severe, may include laryngeal edema
- GI effects, including vomiting and diarrhea

Treatment

- Thoroughly decontaminate casualties as soon as possible.
- **Observe casualties for at least 8 hours.**
- Skin—Administer soothing ointments for skin injury.
- Eyes—Rinse eyes with large amounts of water or Normal Saline (NS) for 5–10 minutes.
- Gastrointestinal—Administer atropine (0.4 mg–0.6 mg) or Ondansetron (4 mg) to relieve early vomiting.
- Neutropenia—Administer filgrastim if the patient has an absolute neutrophil count less than 500/mcL.
- Airways—**Mustard damage to airways is dose-dependent.** As a general rule, early-onset airway symptoms suggest a significant amount of inhaled mustard, although more serious effects will not manifest until hours later.

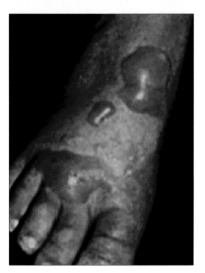

108

Lewisite

Lewisite is a vesicant that, like sulfur mustard, causes damage to skin, the eyes, and the airways by direct contact. **Unlike mustard, Lewisite causes pain rapidly on contact.** Lewisite is an oily colorless liquid and has the scent of geraniums. Lewisite is more volatile (vapor pressure = 0.58 mm Hg at 25°C) than sulfur mustard (vapor pressure = 0.11 mm Hg at 25°C). The exact mechanism by which Lewisite causes tissue damage is unclear.

Clinical Effects

Lewisite damages the tissue it encounters first, often the skin, the eyes, and the airway. Effects are noticeable far more quickly than with mustard. Exposure will cause:

- Damage and blistering of the skin within minutes
- Eye irritation and lid edema
- Airway damage, laryngeal edema, and non-cardiogenic pulmonary edema

Treatment

- Employ the same procedures as with sulfur mustard, except filgrastim is not necessary because neutropenia is not commonly caused by Lewisite.
- Administer British-Anti-Lewisite (BAL) IM if available (usually in a hospital setting).

Hydrogen Cyanide

Hydrogen cyanide has a long history as a deadly poison because it causes death within minutes of exposure. Under temperate conditions, hydrogen cyanide evaporates quickly to form a vapor (boiling point = 25.6°C; vapor pressure = 742 mm Hg at 25°C). **The form of cyanide most likely to be used in a terrorist attack is hydrogen cyanide.** Hydrogen cyanide is the only cyanide considered in this chapter.

Cyanide inhibits cytochrome-c oxidase, which is present in cells. Cytochrome-c oxidase metabolizes oxygen and produces the energy needed for cells to live. When this enzyme is inhibited, the cell cannot produce adequate energy and soon dies. Before death, the cell changes to anaerobic metabolism, causing lactic acidosis.

FIELD OBSERVATION

Lewisite has the scent of geraniums.

LEWISITE TREATMENT

- Treat Lewisite exposure the same as mustard exposure.
- BAL is the specific antidote for Lewisite.

FIELD OBSERVATION

There are two distinctive findings reported in some cyanide casualties.

- Cherry-red skin
- The odor of bitter almonds on the victim's breath

These findings are not *pathognomonic* (diagnostic in themselves) and not always apparent.

The cells in the central nervous system (CNS) are most sensitive to lack of oxygen, and most signs and symptoms from hydrogen cyanide poisoning are of CNS origin.

Clinical Effects
Characteristic clinical effects occur quickly after inhaling a large amount of hydrogen cyanide:

- Transient rapid and deep breathing for about five breaths, starting about 15 seconds after inhalation
- Loss of consciousness and convulsions after approximately 30 seconds
- Breathing stops in 3-5 minutes
- Heart stops in 5-8 minutes

Lesser amounts of inhaled hydrogen cyanide cause anxiety, agitation, vertigo, nausea, and muscular trembling before unconsciousness, apnea, and cardiac arrest. **Antidotes are very effective for hydrogen cyanide casualties.**

Treatment
The following measures are very effective for casualties, whether breathing or not, who still have a pulse.

- Administer oxygen (use bag-valve mask if casualty is not breathing).
- As soon as possible, administer components of the Cyanide Antidote Kit or Hydroxocobalamin.
- The Cyanide Antidote Kit may contain:
    o An ampule of Amyl Nitrite—administer via bag-valve mask for 30 seconds out of every minute until IV is placed
    o 300 mg Sodium Nitrite IV
    o Sodium Thiosulfate (12.5 g in 50 mL) IV
- If symptoms persist, <u>repeat</u> above at half-dose.
- Keep casualties supine after nitrite administration because nitrites cause orthostatic hypotension.
- Hydroxocobalamin 5 g IV is the alternative to administering the Cyanide Antidote Kit.

TREATMENT ALERT!

In contrast to a convulsing nerve agent victim, a convulsing cyanide casualty has:
- Normal sized pupils
- Normal amounts of secretions
- Few or no fasciculations

TREATMENT ALERT!

A casualty who is conscious, talking, and continues to improve will probably not need cyanide antidotes.

Pulmonary Agents

These gases include agents causing pulmonary edema. The best known of these is phosgene, an agent used in World War I that is now widely used in industry. While other compounds in this category such as chlorine have been less well studied, the same management principles apply.

Phosgene (boiling point = 8.2°C) and chlorine (boiling point = -34°C) are gases and enter the body through inhalation. Phosgene and chlorine cause pulmonary edema by damaging the thin membrane between the capillaries of the lung and the *alveoli* (air sacs), the alveolar-capillary membrane.

When inhaled, phosgene and chlorine travel to the alveoli where they break down the alveolar-capillary membrane. Plasma from the blood then leaks through the disrupted membranes into the alveoli, filling these air sacs with fluid. **The pulmonary edema caused by phosgene and chlorine eventually causes dry-land drowning to the point that the casualty can become hypoxic and apneic.**

Clinical Effects

Initially, victims may complain of a transient irritation of the eyes, nose, and throat immediately after exposure, depending on the pulmonary agent's concentration and the victim's duration of exposure. Major respiratory effects do not appear until 2-24 hours after exposure, depending on the amount inhaled. The shorter the time until onset of effects, the greater the damage will be.

The casualty will notice the following:

- A mild shortness of breath that increases in severity over hours
- Coughing that eventually produces clear, frothy sputum due to pulmonary edema may occur in 2-24 hours

Treatment

A casualty with onset of pulmonary edema later than 6 hours of exposure will probably not die given adequate medical care. However, a casualty with onset of pulmonary edema within 4-6 hours of exposure has a poor prognosis, even with optimal care.

- The casualty must avoid all exertion.
- Ventilate as needed.

FIELD OBSERVATION

Phosgene has the scent of freshly cut grass or hay.

TREATMENT ALERT!

It is imperative that lung agent casualties avoid all exertion. Any activity—even walking—will worsen damage to the lungs.

Incapacitating Agents

Evidence suggests the Russian military used a mixture of halothane gas and aerosolized *carfentanil* (an analogue of the popular synthetic opioid analgesic fentanyl, with a quantitative potency approximately 10,000 times that of morphine and 100 times that of fentanyl) to incapacitate Chechen rebels holding civilian hostages in a Moscow theater in 2002. BZ (3-quinuclidinyl benzilate), another incapacitating agent, has marked anticholinergic effects.

Clinical Effects

- Carfentanil produces a typical opioid toxidrome triad with decreased pupil size, decreased level of consciousness, and decreased respirations.

- BZ produces a typical anticholinergic toxidrome with the patient, "red as a beet, dry as a bone, mad as a hatter, blind as a bat, and hot as Hades."

Treatment

- Remove clothing and decontaminate the skin with water and a liquid skin detergent.

- Supply oxygen and ventilation as needed.

- Administer naloxone for opioid (e.g., carfentanil) toxicity.

- Consider physostigmine for anticholinergic delirium caused by BZ.

Riot Control Agents

Riot control agents, also known as tear gases or lacrimators, are usually dispersed as powders suspended in liquids. Injuries from riot control agents are generally not life-threatening, and medical assistance is less commonly sought after exposure to these agents.

Clinical Effects

- Pain, tearing, and redness of the eyes, with chemical conjunctivitis
- Burning of nose and throat, sneezing, and rhinorrhea
- Shortness of breath, bronchospasm, and respiratory distress can occur, especially in asthmatic patients or those with chronic obstructive pulmonary disease
- Tingling and burning sensation in exposed skin, skin erythema

Treatment

- Irrigate eyes copiously with water or NS.
- Wash skin with large amounts of cool water and a liquid skin detergent.
- Administer bronchodilators for bronchospasm.

Decontamination

Decontamination is the process by which a chemical agent is removed or the amount decreased so that it is no longer a hazard.

There are two major goals of the decontamination of casualties:

- To reduce or prevent injury to the casualty. To be most effective, this must be done within minutes of exposure to a solid or liquid agent.

- Before the casualty is decontaminated, all responders in contact with the casualty must wear appropriate protective equipment to prevent secondary contamination of rescue personnel, medical responders, transport units, and the receiving medical facility.

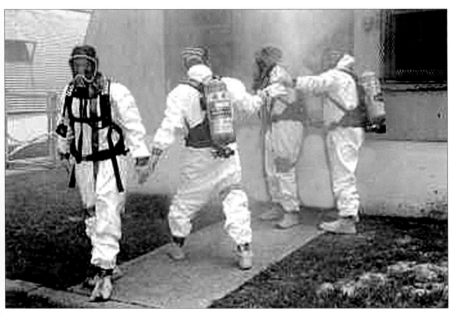

Fig.11.7 Decontamination team equipped with personal protective equipment (PPE), Courtesy of Drug Enforcement Agency (DEA)

STANDARD PRACTICE:

DECONTAMINATION

A dilute (0.5%) sodium hypochlorite bleach solution has been used by the military for skin decontamination. Most civilian EMS units now use large amounts of water and a liquid skin detergent for decontamination.

Decontamination is done in the warm zone, the area that separates the "hot zone" (the contaminated area) from the "cold" zone (free of contamination).

Summary

AGENT	Signs and Symptoms	Decontamination	Emergency Care
Nerve Agents	Small Vapor Exposure: • Miosis • Rhinorrhea Large Vapor Exposure: • Loss of consciousness • Convulsions • Apnea • Flaccid paralysis Small Liquid Exposure: • Localized sweating • Localized fasciculations • Nausea • Vomiting • Diarrhea • Weakness Large Liquid Exposure: • Loss of consciousness • Convulsions • Apnea • Flaccid paralysis	A dilute (0.5%) sodium hypochlorite (bleach) solution has been used by the military for skin decontamination. Most civilian EMS units now use large amounts of water and a liquid skin detergent for this purpose.	• Ventilation • Suction copious secretions from airways • Atropine • Pralidoxime (2-PAM) • Diazepam autoinjector for convulsions
Vesicants	• Erythema • Blisters or wheals • Conjunctivitis • Upper respiratory distress • Pain is delayed with sulfur mustard • Pain occurs rapidly with Lewisite	Thoroughly flush with water and a liquid skin detergent. This must be done immediately after exposure to be maximally effective for sulfur mustard.	• Immediate decontamination • Observe for at least 8 hours • Symptomatic management of lesions (later) • Filgrastim for neutropenia with an absolute neutrophil count less than 500/microliter due to sulfur mustard (in hospital)

Hydrogen cyanide	Large Exposure:
	• Loss of consciousness
	• Convulsions
	• Apnea
	• Cardiac arrest
		Vapor
		• None
		
		Liquid
		• Remove clothing
		• Use large amounts of water and a liquid skin detergent for skin decontamination.
			• Ventilation with O_2
			• Cyanide Antidote Kit
			   o An amp Amyl Nitrite via bag-valve mask
			   o IV Sodium Nitrite
			   o IV Sodium Thiosulfate
			   Or
			   o Hydroxocobalamin IV

Summary (Continued)

AGENT	Signs and Symptoms	Decontamination	Emergency Care
Pulmonary Agents	<u>Initial Signs:</u> • Eye and airway irritation <u>Later Effects:</u> • Pulmonary edema with shortness of breath, cough, and clear, frothy sputum	• None usually	• Termination of exposure • O_2 as needed • No physical activity
Incapacitating Agents	<u>Carfentanil decreases:</u> • Pupil size • Level of consciousness • Respirations <u>BZ causes anticholinergic effects:</u> • Red as a beet • Dry as a bone • Mad as a hatter • Blind as a bat • Hot as Hades	• Thoroughly flush with water and a liquid skin detergent.	• Naloxone for carfentanil toxicity • Administer bronchodilators for bronchospasm.
Riot Control Agents	• Burning eyes, airway, and skin • Respiratory discomfort, bronchospasm	• Fresh air • Flush eyes with water or NS • Flush skin with cool water and a liquid skin detergent	• None usually needed

KEY POINTS

Treatment areas should be upwind and uphill from the contamination site.

Life-saving treatments, such as the IM administration of antidotes, can be done in the Hot Zone by personnel wearing appropriate protective gear.

Medical responders must utilize the appropriate personal protective equipment when triaging and decontaminating "contaminated" victims.

Time is of the essence in the treatment of most chemical agent casualties.

Radioactive Agents

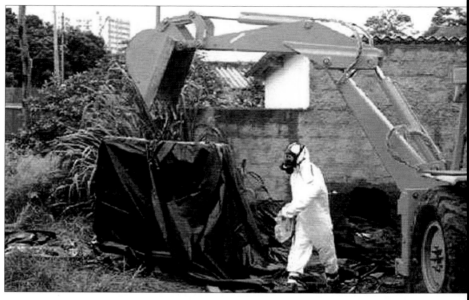

Fig.12.1 Disgarded radiation device, Goiania, Brazil (1987), Courtesy of International Atomic Energy Agency (IAEA)

CASE SCENARIO

In September, 1987, a radiation accident occurred in the city of Goiania in central Brazil. A cancer treatment machine containing Cesium 137 had been abandoned when a medical clinic moved to a new location. The discarded machine was in a building in downtown Goiania for over a year until two men found the machine and sold it to a local junkyard. Workers at the junkyard, unaware of the potential hazard, dismantled the machine, releasing the Cesium that was still active inside the device. The half-life of Cesium is 30.17 years (Centers for Disease Control). Fascinated by the glowing stone and unaware that the object was emitting radiation, the workers distributed pieces to friends and relatives. Four individuals died from exposure and over 100,000 had to be monitored for contamination. 249 individuals were found to have significant levels of radioactive material in or on their body. The International Atomic Energy Agency called it "one of the world's worst radiological incidents."

Introduction

Many different disaster scenarios involve the uncontrolled release of dangerous radioactive materials. Disasters involving release of radioactive material may be unintentional (accidents) or intentional (terrorism).

Release of radioactive material would likely involve one of four scenarios, listed in order of most-to-least devastating, but, fortunately, least-to-most likely.

1. Detonation of a nuclear device—nuclear explosion
2. Meltdown of a nuclear reactor—melting of the nuclear fuel within a reactor with release of radioactive materials into the environment
3. Dispersal of material through use of conventional explosives—a radiological dispersal device (RDD) or "dirty bomb"
4. Non-explosive dispersal of nuclear material

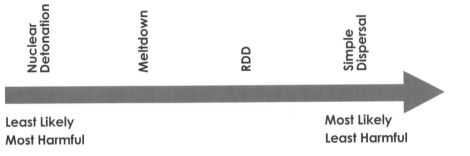

Nuclear Detonation   Meltdown   RDD   Simple Dispersal

Least Likely
Most Harmful

Most Likely
Least Harmful

Principles of Ionizing Radiation

Radiation is everywhere. Sunlight and radar are forms of non-ionizing radiation. Cell phones use non-ionizing radiation to transmit our conversations.

Ionizing radiation is radiation that can injure living tissue by transferring energy to vital cell components. Ionizing radiation is a natural part of our environment. Everyone is continuously exposed to a small amount of ionizing radiation, called *background radiation*. Sources of background radiation are both natural and man-made.

Sources of Radiation Exposure

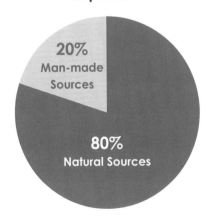

20% Man-made Sources

80% Natural Sources

Fig. 12.2

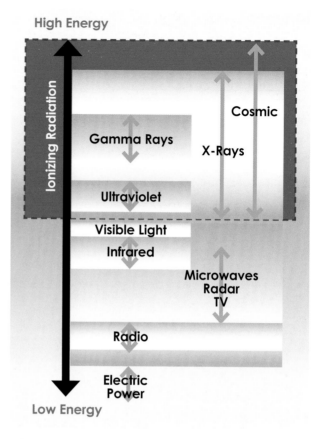

Fig 12.3 Types of ionizing and non-ionizing radiation

Types of Ionizing Radiation
There are two types of ionizing radiation: electromagnetic (wave) radiation and particle radiation. Ionizing electromagnetic radiation consists of gamma rays and x-rays. Particle radiation consists of alpha particles, beta particles, and neutrons.

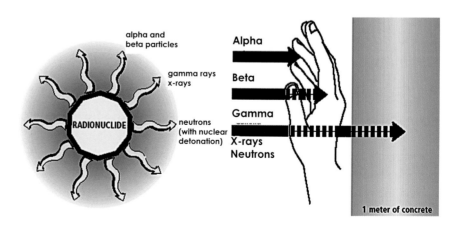

Fig 12.4 Penetrating power of ionizing radiation

Types of Ionizing Radiation

Type of Ionizing Radiation	Description	Dispersal	Physical Harm Caused
Alpha particles (α)	Large positively charged radiation particles containing 2 protons and 2 neutrons	Particle fallout—can only travel centimeters from source in air	• Not an external hazard • Highly destructive if the source is inhaled, injected, or absorbed through an open wound • Usually causes cellular death in immediate tissue area
Beta particles (β)	Small negatively charged particles (electrons) that are released from the decaying nucleus of a radioactive substance	Particle fallout—can travel only several meters in the air	• Skin is vulnerable to acute injury ("Beta Burns") • Lens of the eye vulnerable to cataract formation • Source can be ingested and absorbed through open wounds • Potentially carcinogenic to internal organs • Effect is dose dependent
Gamma rays (γ)	Very energetic form of electromagnetic radiation that passes through body tissues and deposits energy in tissues	Wave radiation—can travel kilometers in air at the speed of light	• Internal and external irradiation hazard • Acute and/or delayed injury • Carcinogenic effect depending on dose
Neutrons	Uncharged particles that pass through body tissues and deposit their energy in tissue	Result of nuclear fission only—can travel many meters in air	• Internal hazard through collision with molecules in tissue • Captured by atoms in tissue and subsequently release gamma radiation

Biological Effects of Ionizing Radiation

Ionizing radiation transfers energy to cells in the body. If the radiation is strong enough, the cell will be killed or undergo apoptosis (programmed cell death). Less severe radiation exposure and resultant damage may exceed the cell's ability to repair itself or leave permanent alterations in the cell's functioning or genetic material (e.g., predispose to development of cancer).

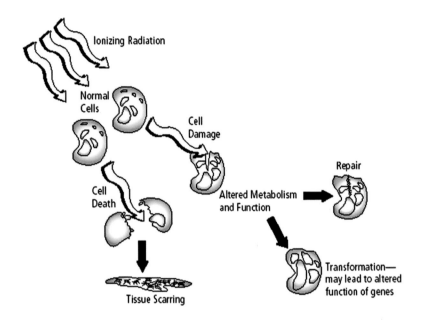

12.5 Biological effects on cells

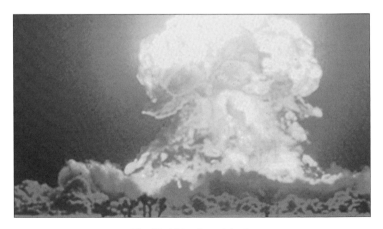

Fig. 12.6 Nuclear blast

There are two general types of radiation exposure, which may occur alone or simultaneously:

- **External irradiation (radiation exposure)**
    - o Whole body irradiation
    - o Localized irradiation
- **Contamination (radiation debris)**
    - o External contamination
    - o Internal contamination

External Irradiation

- External irradiation occurs when all or part of the body is exposed to electromagnetic radiation—gamma rays or x-rays—from an external source. The degree of injury depends upon the dose of radiation received. (Dose = exposure time X exposure rate.)

- During exposure, radiation can pass completely through the body, or its energy can be absorbed by body tissues.

- Accidental exposure to a high-radiation source exposes the whole body, but exposure to the extremities, particularly the hands and fingers, is usually the greatest, as they will probably be closest to the source and will have minimal shielding.

Contamination

External Contamination

- **External contamination occurs when radioactive debris (sometimes referred to as fallout) is deposited on the body and clothing.**

- This radioactive material can exist in dust particle form. Particles may be suspended in air and may then be deposited on skin and clothing.

- Contamination of the skin and hair by radioactive materials can be removed by thorough surface cleaning. Generally, external contamination is not a serious medical problem as long as the material and contaminated clothing are removed quickly. Care must be taken to prevent inadvertent internal contamination by external material on clothing or skin.

RISK ALERT!

Radioactive contamination is dangerous because it can continue to irradiate the parts of the body it is near.

Prior to decontamination, a contaminated patient does not present an immediate irradiation hazard to medical personnel who utilize normal barrier protection.

Internal Contamination

- **Internal contamination occurs when radioactive materials are inhaled, ingested, or absorbed through open wounds.** The assessment and management of internal contamination is more difficult than for external contamination and is not an emergent condition.

- Radioactive materials may become concentrated in particular tissues, resulting in high-intensity local exposures.

- Radioactive iodine is concentrated in the thyroid gland in the same way as non-radioactive iodine. Consequently, the thyroid gland is exposed to radiation injury. Radioactive iodine can be inhaled or ingested.

Radiation Threat Scenarios

Nuclear Detonations

Two basic differences exist between nuclear and conventional explosions: size of the explosion and presence of radiation and radioactive debris. **Nuclear detonations cause three types of injuries: blast, thermal, and radiation.**

Blast Injuries

Blast injuries are caused by the overpressure wave that travels out from Ground Zero (detonation area) at several hundred miles per hour, causing primary blast-pressure injuries as it expands.

Thermal Injuries

Flash Burns

Flash burns can occur in all those directly exposed to the infrared wave pulse.

- Casualties are burned on the side facing the explosion, with light-color clothing reflecting the infrared wave and dark clothing absorbing it, causing "pattern burns."

- Eye injuries, especially to the chorioretinal areas, are caused by both the sudden exposures to high-intensity visible light and the infrared radiation of a detonation.

- Looking directly at the flash would cause retinal burns. Flash blindness would occur with peripheral observation of a brilliant flash of intense light energy, for example, a fireball.

Flame Burns

The firestorm caused by the infrared wave would result in typical flame burns as well as closed space fire-associated injuries.

Components of a nuclear detonation

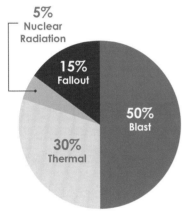

Fig 12.7

FIELD OBSERVATION

The thermal radiation emitted by a nuclear detonation causes burns in two ways:

- Flash burns
- Flame burns

Flammable materials will ignite and burn for hours after the initial blast. Casualties will suffer:

- Toxic gas injuries from burning plastics and other materials
- Superheated air inhalation burns
- Steam burns from ruptured pipes
- All other large conflagration-type injuries

Any object between a person and the infrared wave pulse and the resulting fireball will provide a measure of protection. Close to the fireball, however, the intense thermal output will preclude survival.

Radiation Injuries

A nuclear detonation will result in extremely high dose rates from radiation during the initial 60 seconds (irradiation by gamma rays and neutrons) at Ground Zero. Fission products (residual radionuclides and daughters) will be present in the fallout area relatively close to Ground Zero. These will be deposited in areas outside the blast area, as determined by atmospheric winds immediately after the detonation. This early fallout will emit alpha and beta particles and intense gamma radiation, and it will cause radiation injury to persons who do not rapidly evacuate the contaminated area. If a nuclear weapon has been "laced" with some materials, e.g., strontium, the resultant fallout could be highly radioactive for decades.

RISK ALERT!

The severity of radiation illness is dependent upon the dose of radiation received.

DOSE = EXPOSURE TIME X DOSE RATE.

Meltdown of a Nuclear Reactor

Nuclear power plant accidents are real threats as illustrated by the Fukushima accident in Japan. An earthquake severely damaged the nuclear power plant with extensive contamination of the adjacent region.

Reactors operate at high temperatures, contain a specific mixture of radioactive elements, and produce all radiation types. Several problems must occur simultaneously for a nuclear meltdown to affect the general population:

- The core must dramatically overheat, causing the nuclear fuel to melt. The subsequent control loss would release tremendous amounts of radiation. This scenario can occur when there is a catastrophic failure of the core's cooling systems or when the reactor protection system fails to shut down the reactor in the face of a catastrophic problem.

- If a core meltdown occurs, large amounts of radioactive materials would only be released to the external environment if there were also a major failure of the containment structure, such as an overpressure relief failure within the containment structure or a failure of the containment isolation systems, lines, and valves to close. The reactor at Chernobyl had no containment system.

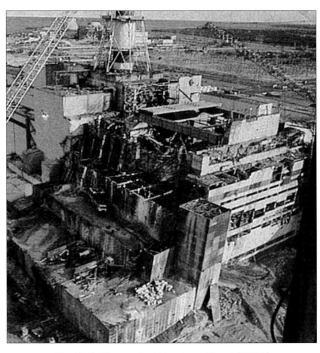

Fig. 12.8 Chernobyl Nuclear Plant (1986)

TREATMENT ALERT!

Iodine pills, often provided to people living close to a nuclear power plant in case of an accident, are effective only as prophylaxis against the effects of radioactive iodine on the thyroid gland.

They provide no protection against any other radioactive material.

- Coolant system leaks could also release smaller amounts of radioactivity.

- Radioactive substances released by an operating nuclear power plant failure would include radioactive iodine and noble gases.

Damage to spent (but still radioactive) fuel rods would produce radiation similar to that produced by a radiological dispersal device (RDD), far less than would occur in a core meltdown.

Radiological Dispersal Device (RDD)

A RDD is any device that purposefully disseminates radioactive material across an area without a nuclear detonation. An RDD ("dirty bomb") generally uses an explosive agent (such as TNT or a plastic explosive) to disseminate its radioactive materials. The radioactive material dispersed can originate from any location that uses radioactive sources, including:

- A nuclear waste processor
- A nuclear power plant
- A university research facility
- A medical radiotherapy clinic
- An industrial complex

Radiological dispersal devices kill or injure those closest to the explosion by mechanical trauma and generate a cloud of radioactive materials, subsequently contaminating victims and medical responders. The larger the explosive, the wider the radioactive material will be spread, but the smaller the dose-rate at any given point. An RDD does not create more radioactive material; it simply scatters the material that is already there.

Internal contamination among persons remaining in the area is an RDD's prime radioactive danger. The contaminated ground areas can be readily detected with conventional radiacs. Areas where the point dose-rate exceeds the allowable legal limits for the general public must be decontaminated before allowing unmonitored entry.

Simple Radiological Devices

A simple radiological device deliberately spreads radioactive materials without an explosion.

- The placement of a Cobalt 60 radioisotope in a public place would expose many individuals to varying radiation levels. Individual injury levels would be determined by the exposure of the individual as delineated by physical proximity and the exposure duration.

RDD DEFINED

A RDD is a conventional explosive designed to spread radioactive material. An RDD does not cause a nuclear explosion.

Emergency Management of Radiation Casualties

The extent of exposure will vary according to the type of ionizing radiation involved in the incident. Charged particles (alphas and betas) are easily stopped. Neutrons and gamma rays easily penetrate body tissues as well as glass and plastic. Although medical providers may not know the exact type of ionizing radiation released in a specific incident, certain general principles are known.

THE CARDINAL RULE OF PROTECTION AGAINST RADIATION IS TIME, DISTANCE, AND SHIELDING.

Time

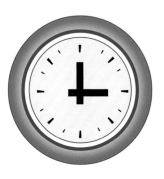

Time
The shorter the amounts of time you spend near the radiation source, the less radiation exposure you receive.

- Medical responders should limit the time they are exposed to a radioactive source by working in short, rotating shifts as directed by the radiation safety officer.

Distance

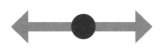

Distance
The farther away you are from a radiation source, the less exposure you receive. Radiation diminishes with the square of the distance from the source.

- Medical responders should deploy from the cold zone, or behind a protective barrier, and return immediately to a safe area when their shift is finished. The amount of exposure each responder will be allowed to accumulate must be determined prior to his/her deployment.

Shielding

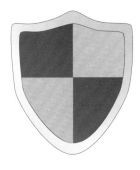

Shielding
Increasing the shielding around a radiation source—or around you—decreases your exposure.

- **Medical responders must wear individual dosimeters and personal protection garments capable of preventing contact with, inhalation of, and ingestion of radioactive materials.** After rotating into a hot zone, personnel should return to an area behind protective barriers as soon as possible, and their individual exposure recorded.

Medical Effects of Ionizing Radiation

There are several effects of ionizing radiation on the body. The degree of effect depends on the type of the radiation and the dose of exposure.

- **Focal tissue damage and necrosis** result from localized exposure, i.e., "Beta Burns". These only appear to be burns, but are really intense areas of local tissue injury. They will evolve over time and may take months to heal.

- **Acute radiation sickness** is the result of whole-body exposure.

- **Long-term effects** (weeks, months, and years to decades) include pneumonitis, cataracts, thyroid cancer, and a higher incidence of leukemia and certain other cancers.

Focal Burns and Necrosis

<u>Localized</u> exposure to radiation can result in various skin changes, depending upon the dose of radiation received. This is not a total body dose; it is the local tissue dose from a source situated close to the skin.

- >3 Gy (300 rad)—*epilation* (hair loss)

- >6 Gy (600 rad)—erythema

- >10 Gy (1,000 rad)—*desquamation* (flaking off of skin)

- >20 Gy (2,000 rad)—necrosis

These changes in the skin, with the exception of necrosis, appear similar to severe sunburn or chemical burns, but should be treated more like frostbite. Tissue loss will be progressive, and areas that initially appear hyperemic may progress over time to necrosis. Debridement must be extremely cautious.

- The amount of radiation you absorb has been measured in rad.

- The biological effect of this radiation has been measured in rem.

- These effects are now measured in newer international units, the gray (Gy) and sievert (Sv).

  o **100 rad = 1 Gy**

  o **100 rem = 1 Sv**

Acute Radiation Syndrome (ARS)

ARS is a group of clinical subsyndromes that develop acutely (within several seconds to several days) after exposure to penetrating ionizing radiation above average whole-body doses of 1 Gy (100 rad). ARS affects different systems, depending on the total dose of radiation received.

- Lower doses predominantly damage the hematopoietic system.

- Increasing doses damage the gastrointestinal system, the cardiovascular system, and the central nervous system in that order.

- **The higher the exposure, the earlier symptoms will appear, and the worse the prognosis is.**

- A whole-body exposure of 5 Gy (500 rad) has a mortality rate of 100% due to bone marrow failure and gastrointestinal damage unless appropriate medical treatment is provided.

- A whole-body exposure of 10 Gy (1,000 rads) is the approximate maximum total-body dose potentially survivable with the best and most aggressive medical therapy available. Open wounds in conjunction with radiation injury will dramatically decrease survival probability.

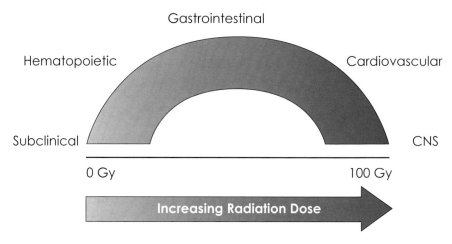

Fig 12.9 Acute Radiation Syndrome

ARS progresses through four stages:

- **Prodromal phase**
- **Latent phase**
- **Manifest illness phase**
- **Recovery or death phase**

128

Prodromal Phase

- Depending on the total amount of radiation absorbed, casualties may experience a variety of symptoms, including:

    o Appetite loss

    o Nausea

    o Vomiting

    o Fatigue

    o Diarrhea

- After high doses of radiation, prostration, fever, respiratory difficulty, and increased excitability may develop.
- **The earlier the symptoms appear, the worse the prognosis.**
- It is important to note that nausea and vomiting may be due to anxiety and not to radiation exposure.

Prodromal Symptoms, Time of Onset, Radiation Dose, and Eventual Clinical Effects in ARS

Symptoms (Prodromal Phase)	Time of Onset of Symptoms	Approximate Whole-Body Radiation Dose	Eventual Physiologic Effects (Manifest Illness Phase)
Nausea, vomiting (due to radiation alone)	Within first 48 hours	1 Gy 100 rad	Decrease in white cells and platelets
Nausea, vomiting	Within first 24 hours	2 Gy 200 rad	Marked decrease in white cells and platelets (hematopoietic syndrome)
Nausea, vomiting, diarrhea	Within first 12 hours (8 hours for diarrhea)	4 Gy 400 rad	Gastrointestinal damage 50% mortality in the absence of treatment
Nausea, vomiting, diarrhea	Within 5 minutes	10 –30 Gy 1,000 –3,000 rad	Severe gastrointestinal damage (gastrointestinal syndrome) Very poor prognosis
CNS effects, mental status changes	Within minutes	>30 Gy >3,000 rad	Severe CNS damage, coupled with cardiovascular collapse (neurovascular syndrome) Lethal

Latent Phase

- Following recovery from the prodromal phase, the exposed individual will be relatively symptom-free, but easily fatigued.
- **Depending on the exposure level, the latent phase will last longer (corresponding to less exposure), or shorter (corresponding to more exposure).**
    o The latent phase is longest preceding the bone marrow depression of the hematopoietic syndrome, lasting between 2 and 6 weeks.
    o The latent period is somewhat shorter prior to the gastrointestinal syndrome, lasting from a few days to a week.
    o The latent phase is shortest preceding the neurovascular syndrome, lasting only a matter of hours.
- **A reduced lymphocyte count can occur within 48 hours and is a clinical indicator of the radiation severity.**
    o >1,200—good prognosis
    o 300-1,200—potentially lethal
    o <300—critical
- Other symptoms, such as weakness, hair loss, and weight loss, may occur as well.

Manifest Illness

- This phase presents with the clinical symptoms associated with the major organ system injured (marrow, intestinal, neurovascular) described in the chart on the preceding page.

Death or Recovery Phase

- Persons exposed to >10 Gy (1,000 rad) of radiation will generally die within 72 hours without medical care.
- Casualties exposed to 4-10 Gy (400-1,000 rad) are likely to die unless medically treated.
- Casualties exposed to less than 4 Gy (400 rad) will generally recover, given effective hematopoietic stimulation as needed and appropriate protection from secondary infection.

Long-term Effects

Long-term stochastic effects of radiation exposure are "all-or-nothing"—either cancer will develop or it will not. Depending upon the damage done to tissue by the ionizing radiation, casualties may have an increased risk of cancer and other manifestations.

Triage of Radiation Casualties

Since the clinical effects of all but the most severe radiation exposures are delayed, the clinical presentation of exposed casualties will be primarily related to conventional injuries sustained in the event that triggers the release of the radioactive material.

- **Trauma triage procedures should be employed, and early closure of simple wounds is mandatory in irradiated casualties.**
- Depending on the severity of the casualty's condition and triage status, decontamination can be done before, during, or after initial stabilization.
- Triage casualties who have received exposure >2 Gy (200 rad) and who require any surgery to treatment immediately.

Decontamination of Radiation Casualties

- Individuals who have been irradiated, i.e., exposed to a source or a radiation blast of gamma rays and neutrons, are not contaminated and, therefore, do not need decontamination.
- **For those externally contaminated with radioactive material, the removal of clothing usually eliminates more than 90% of the contamination.**
- If the casualty has surface contamination and no physical injuries, washing with soap and water provides effective decontamination.
- If the contaminated casualty has substantial physical injuries, the casualty should be stabilized before decontamination is performed.
- The skin is an important barrier to radioactive material and should not be abraded during decontamination. Skin should be gently washed, not scrubbed.

RISK ALERT!

Know the limitations of your radiation detection devices! Many radiation detectors (radiacs) measure only beta and gamma radiation.

Emergency Treatment

- Many acute radiation exposures without associated physical injuries do not require medical attention within the first few hours of exposure. Emergency treatment should focus on physical injuries to casualties that may be life-threatening.
- If a casualty is suspected of having received a dose of >2 Gy (200 rad), every effort must be made to close every wound, cover every burn, reduce every fracture, and perform any and all surgeries within the first 48 hours. After 48 hours, all surgical interventions must be delayed for 2-3 months due to hematopoietic depression and inadequate wound healing. Necessary surgery during this window will result in markedly increased morbidity and mortality.

Emergency Surgery	No Surgery Hematopoietic Recovery	Surgery Permitted
24-48 hours	3 months	After 3 months

Special Issues

- The incident commander will determine how much radiation exposure will be allowable for individual responders and will set the maximum allowable _cumulative_ dose.

- All responders must be equipped with direct-reading individual dosimeters that cannot be reset by the individual. Readings from these dosimeters must be recorded as frequently as possible to ensure individual exposures do not inadvertently exceed the maximum allowable dose.

- THERE ARE NO EXCEPTIONS TO THIS RULE. When ANY responder's total dose exposure reaches the maximum allowable dose as set by the safety officer, the responder must leave the site immediately. The responder cannot return until all remediation activities are complete, and the site is opened to the general public.

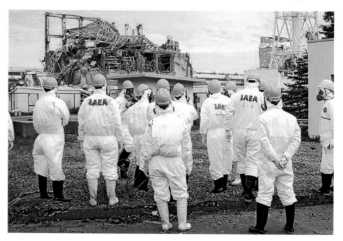

*Fig.12.10 Fukushima nuclear accident (2012),
Courtesy of IAEA*

Summary

Radiation accidents, unintentional or intentional, pose significant challenges to medical providers. The severity of radiation illness is based upon radiation dose and exposure time. Contamination with radioactive materials is usually not life-threatening, and decontamination procedures are straightforward. Decontamination should be done as soon as possible but does not require the same urgency as chemical decontamination. Removing clothing will significantly decrease the amount of external contamination.

KEY POINTS

 Medical providers should assume both external and internal contamination of victims when responding to disasters involving radioactive agents.

 Acute radiation syndrome occurs after whole-body exposure to radioactive agents.

 It is important to know the limitations of radiation detection devices.

Blast Injuries

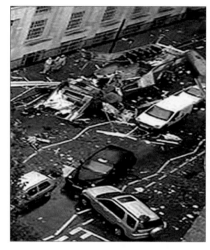 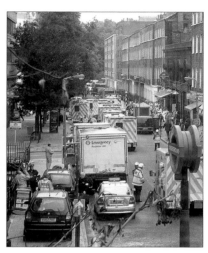

Figs.13.1, 13.2 London Bombing (2005)

CASE SCENARIO

London and its public transport system became the target of terrorist attacks on the morning of July 7, 2005. In a series of coordinated attacks, four suicide bombers detonated explosive devices at various locations in the London transport system during the busy morning rush hour. Three of the bombs exploded in underground trains across the city and one on a double-decker bus in central London. Fifty-two (52) individuals and 4 suicide bombers were killed in the attacks and more than 700 victims injured. The explosions were the result of homemade organic peroxide-based devices contained in rucksacks. Bony fragments from other victims (or possibly the bombers) were found embedded as biological foreign bodies within the soft tissues in several victims.

Introduction

Blast injuries are multi-system, life-threatening injuries that may be caused by many types of disasters. Explosions and bombings, especially those related to terrorism, continue to be a significant challenge for medical providers. Victims sustaining blast injuries, whether due to unintentional explosions such as gas pipeline accidents or intentional terrorist bombings, cause complex triage decisions, diagnostic challenges, and disaster management issues. The ability to manage mass casualty incidents due to blasts needs to be stressed in all healthcare systems.

Individuals who have been injured by explosions/blasts have been termed "multi-dimensional" victims due to the mechanisms of blast injury that these patients sustain (primary, secondary, tertiary, and quaternary injuries). Blast injury victims tend to sustain more traumatic injuries and have more varied anatomic locations of injury and greater injury severity scores (ISS) than other trauma victims. The predominant post-explosion injuries among survivors of blasts involve standard penetrating and blunt trauma.

Explosives

Explosives may be classified as high order or high energy (HE) or low order or low energy (LE)). High energy and LE explosives cause different patterns of injury. High energy explosives **detonate** to produce a defining over-pressurization shock wave. LE explosives **deflagrate** to create a subsonic explosion and lack the HE over-pressurization shock wave.

The blast wave (over-pressure component) created by high-order explosives must be distinguished from "blast wind", which is the forced super-heated air flow. Blast wind may be found in both high and low order explosions.

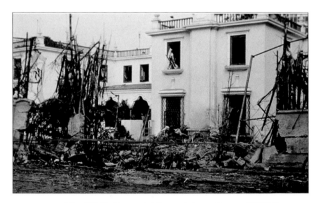

Fig.13.3 Terrorist bombing, Peru (2002)

135

High Order (High Energy) Explosives - Detonation

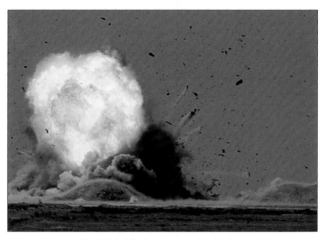

Fig.13.4 High energy explosion

High energy explosives produce a defining supersonic over-pressurization shock wave. The detonation of a high energy explosive causes the instantaneous conversion of the explosive material into highly-pressurized gases and results in a supersonic energy wave. The shock or over-pressure wave travels outward from the center of the explosion. The result of this over-pressurization shock wave causes a "shattering blow" to the immediate surroundings.

Examples of HE explosives are:
C-4
Semtex
Nitroglycerin
Dynamite
Trinitrotoluene (TNT)
Ammonium nitrite-fuel oil (ANFO)

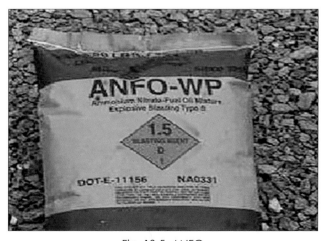

Fig. 13.5 ANFO

The blast or shock waves possess a characteristic termed brisance (shattering effect). *Brisance* is the measure of the rapidity with which an explosive develops its maximum pressure. **This high peak pressure (above atmospheric) is called the peak over-pressure.** As these gases expand outward, they displace the surrounding medium (air or water). The pressure wave propagates rapidly through the surrounding atmosphere. The intensity of the pressure wave declines as the gases expand. The gases slow, and this results in an under-pressure, which returns rapidly to normal atmospheric pressure. This classical waveform is known as a Friedlander wave and describes the pressure changes for a simple blast wave in a free environment, e.g., one without obstacles or constraints.

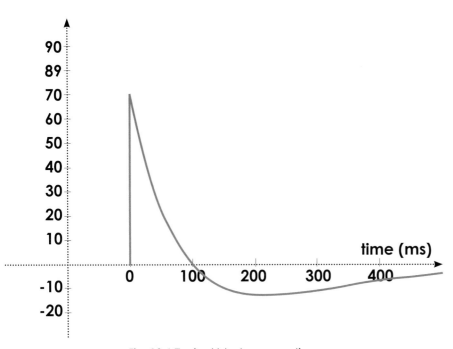

Fig. 13.6 Typical blast-pressure time curve

Low Order (Low Energy) Explosives-Deflagration.

Low energy explosives are classified differently because they lack the self-defining HE over-pressurization wave. **Low energy explosives deflagrate to create a subsonic explosion.** Deflagration is a term describing the subsonic combustion that usually propagates through thermal conductivity. Injuries from LE explosives are due to ballistics (fragmentation), blast wind (not blast wave), and thermal injuries.

Examples of LE explosives include:

- Pipe bombs
- Gunpowder
- Molotov cocktails

Landmines

Military explosive devices follow similar physics to a high energy explosion. The chemical conversion of these explosive devices from a solid into a gaseous state occurs rapidly. Many of these munitions are designed to propel shrapnel and cause significant morbidity and mortality.

In the aftermath of many wars, large numbers of land mines have been left behind, placing the civilian population in harm's way. In many areas of the world, trying to prevent the death and maiming of the civilian population is a public health crisis. Despite a ban on landmine usage, approximately 70 million mines still lay in unmarked minefields in 70 countries throughout the world, with the potential to cause significant injuries and deaths in civilian populations.

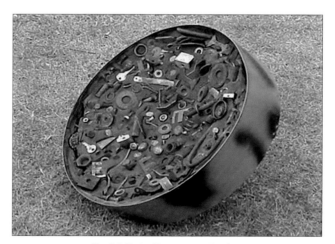

Fig.13.7 Antipersonnel Mine

The lower extremities are at greatest risk from these injuries, resulting in gross deformities, amputations, and fragmentation. Significant soft tissue damage occurs, both from the pressure wave and secondary injuries due to fragmentation. The resultant injuries may also necessitate amputations.

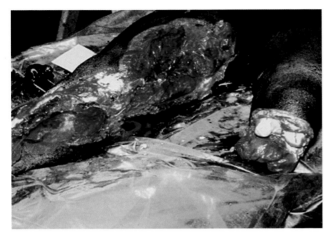

Fig.13.8 Landmine Injury

Improvised Explosive Devices

An improvised explosive device (IED) attack is the use of a "homemade" bomb and/or destructive device to destroy, incapacitate, harass, or distract. IEDs are used by various criminal groups, including terrorists and suicide bombers. IEDs can come in many forms, ranging from small pipe bombs to sophisticated devices capable of causing massive damage and loss of life. IEDs can be carried or delivered in a vehicle; carried, placed, or thrown by a person; delivered in a package; or concealed on the roadside. IED's can be combined with other agents, such as chemical, biological or radioactive agents (dirty bomb).

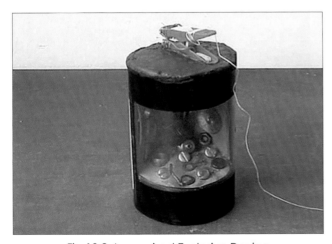

Fig.13.9 Improvised Explosive Device

Severity of Blast Injuries

Open versus Closed Space Blast Injury

The survivability and morbidity from any explosion correlates with whether victims are in an open versus closed space. Multiple studies have demonstrated the significant difference in mortality and morbidity between open versus closed space explosions. The physics and dynamics of blast waves are significantly increased in an "enclosed" environment (e.g., buildings, large vehicles such as buses, mines, etc.). The amplification of the shock wave occurs because the blast waves are reflected off solid objects (walls, floors, ceilings) inside the closed structure. In outdoor explosions, the blast wave dissipates rapidly.

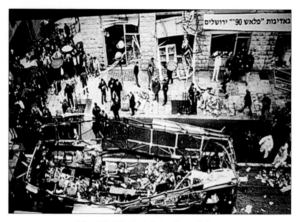

Fig.13.10 Suicide Bombing

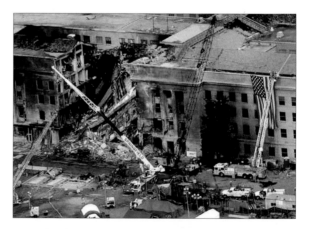

*Fig.13.11 Pentagon terrorist attack (2001),
Courtesy of FEMA*

Underwater Blasts

Special issues need to be considered when blasts occur underwater. Water is a relatively non-compressible medium compared with air; thus, it is a more efficient transmitter. **The lethal radius is increased because the blast waves move at increased speeds and cover more distances.** Underwater explosions are more likely to involve bowel injuries. The thoracic cavity may be partially protected if the chest is not completely immersed, such as when the person is treading water.

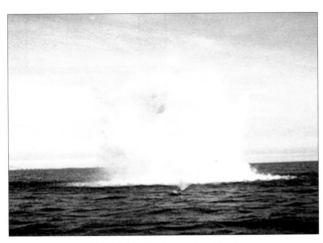

Fig.13.12 Underwater Blast

Mechanisms of Injury

Blast injuries are traditionally divided into four categories depending on the resultant injuries and the presumed mechanisms of injury. These categories are an excellent method to organize the approach to caring for these complex and often critically injured patients. Most blast injuries, however, are a combination of these mechanisms of injury.

Primary Blast Injury (PBI)

Primary blast injuries result from the direct effect of the blast wave (traveling at supersonic speeds) on the body. **Primary blast injuries primarily affect gas-containing organs: the gastrointestinal tract, the lung, and the middle ear.** The proposed mechanisms to explain the injury patterns include the pressure wave differentials that occur at the air-fluid interfaces.

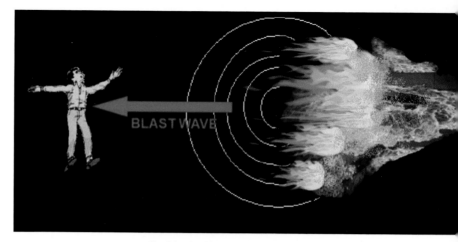

Fig.13.13 Primary Blast Injury (PBI)

The shock wave causes injury via three mechanisms, which can combine to create multiple injuries in the blast victim.

- *Spalling.* When a shock wave moves between tissues of different densities, such as the lung and the ear, the wave changes velocity at the interface. This disrupts the tissue, causing injury.

- *Implosion.* The sudden expansion of gases compressed by the passing shock wave can rupture hollow organs such as the intestines.

- *Shearing.* Shearing is the phenomenon that occurs when tissues of different densities respond to the pressure wave by moving at different speeds in relation to each other.

Pulmonary Injury

The pulmonary system is particularly susceptible to primary blast injury. **The most common lung injury is a pulmonary contusion.** Blast lung (severe pulmonary contusion) is a direct consequence of the HE

> **TREATMENT ALERT!**
>
> Casualties with a mechanism of injury that suggests PBI should be observed for 12-24 hours!

> **Symptoms of Blast Lung Injury**
>
> - DYSPNEA
> - COUGH
> - HEMOPTYSIS
> - CHEST PAIN

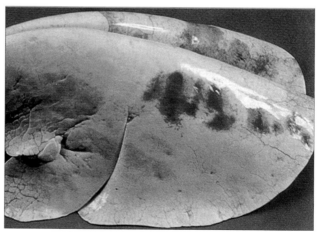

Fig.13.14 Blast Injury to lung

over-pressurization wave. In addition, patients may suffer from a range of other pulmonary injuries ranging from pneumothoraces/hemothoraces to A-V fistulas (source of air emboli).

The clinical management of primary blast injuries to the lung is treated similarly to other causes of pulmonary contusions: treat the underlaying hypoxia with supplemental oxygen. Ensuring adequate ventilation can be a challenge.

The evaluation of a patient who suffers injury to the respiratory system includes routine physical examination, chest radiograph, and pulse oximetry if possible. If the pulmonary symptoms persist despite a normal chest radiograph, further studies are warranted. Chest CT, if available, should be done because blast lung injury and associated complications can be missed on chest radiograph.

Gastrointestinal Injury

Abdominal blast injuries are a significant cause of injury and death. Incidence and clinical presentation of abdominal blast injury will vary significantly depending upon the patient and the nature of the blast. **Underwater blasts carry a significantly greater risk of abdominal injury.** Children are more prone to abdominal injuries due to their unique anatomy.

External examination of the abdomen may reveal no evidence of external trauma (bruising). Upon auscultation and palpation, absent bowel sounds and pain raise the likelihood of barotrauma from

> **TREATMENT ALERT!**
>
> Abdominal ultrasound is an excellent complementary modality to the physical examination. Ultrasound is best for solid organ injury but less reliable for hollow viscus injuries. Abdominal blast injuries may be occult and difficult to diagnose.

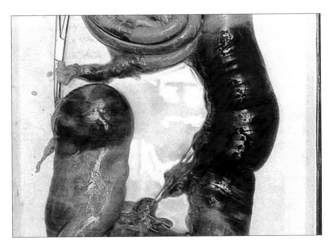

*Fig.13.15 Blast injury to intestine,
Courtesy of Department of Defense*

explosions. Blast injury to the gastrointestinal (GI) tract should be suspected in anyone who has abdominal pain, nausea, vomiting, hematemesis, rectal pain, testicular pain, unexpected hypovolemia, or any finding compatible with an acute abdomen after exposure to an explosion.

Primary blast injury to the GI tract causes a wide spectrum of injuries, ranging from hemorrhage (small petechiae to large hematomas) to mucosal ischemia, bowel wall necrosis, and bowel perforation. The colon and ileocecal region are the visceral organs at greatest risk of intestinal perforation, which is caused by implosion forces rupturing the bowel wall.

Ear Injury

The middle ear is particularly sensitive to stress waves and over-pressure damage. Pressure increases as little as 1 to 8 psi can rupture the human tympanic membrane (TM). **Isolated eardrum rupture alone is not a marker for significant blast injury.** Conversely, significant blast injuries cannot be excluded solely based upon the absence of TM injury. A critical piece of history is whether the patient was wearing protective ear gear (particularly in an industrial situation).

Management of isolated traumatic tympanic perforations can be done as an outpatient. Most of the ruptures heal spontaneously without complication.

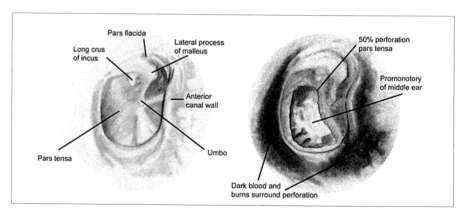

Fig.13.16 Normal and perforated right tympanic membrane, Courtesy of CDC

Secondary Blast Injury

Secondary blast injuries, which can be just as deadly as primary injuries, result from the patient being struck by objects and debris that have been accelerated by the explosion. A favorite practice for terrorists has become packing IEDs and other explosive devices with screws, bolts, nuts, and any other sharp small objects that, when propelled, have deadly consequences. Devastating soft tissue, internal, and orthopedic trauma are frequent from propelled missiles.

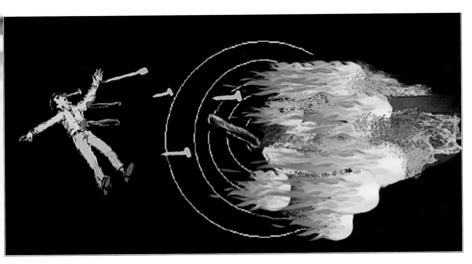

Fig.13.17 Secondary blast Injury

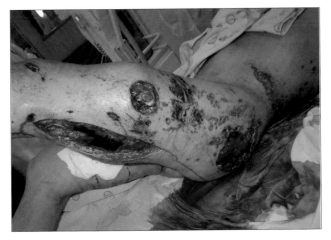

*Fig.13.18 Extensive secondary blast injury to flank
and lower extremity*

145

Tertiary Blast Injury

Tertiary blast injuries result from the victims being thrown from the high winds produced from blast waves. Blast winds may achieve speeds of up to 160 km/hr. Tertiary blast injury casualties sustain major blunt trauma injuries, including traumatic brain injuries, solid organ ruptures, and complex orthopedic injuries. Penetrating trauma can occur when these patients are impaled on objects in the environment. Extrication and immobilization of these patients can be challenging.

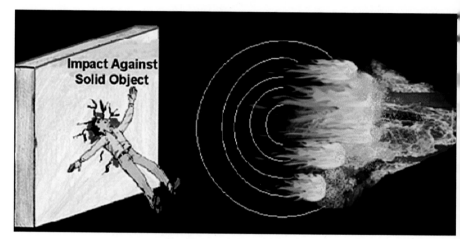

Fig. 13.19 Tertiary blast injury

Quaternary Blast Injury

Miscellaneous or quaternary injuries encompass all other injuries caused by explosives such as burns, crush injuries, and toxic inhalations (carbon monoxide, dust, hot gases). The hazmat aspects of these incidents always need to be considered to protect responders as well as casualties.

Scene Safety

Scene safety is of utmost importance, regardless of the cause of the explosion. The disaster site can be a chaotic environment. In an uncontrolled incident, always be concerned about secondary devices in a potential terrorist event.

Vast numbers of "walking wounded" can lead to a reverse triage effect. Patients with minor injuries present to casualty collection centers or hospitals before the serious casualties arrive, swamping emergency services to the detriment of the severely wounded.

Summary

Blast injuries are significant challenges for disaster providers due to the multi-dimensional nature (primary, secondary, tertiary, and quaternary injuries). Casualties often sustain mixed types of injuries, increasing the diagnostic and treatment challenges.

Category	Mechanism of Injury
Primary Blast Injury	Blast wave
Secondary Blast Injury	Victim struck by flying debris
Tertiary Blast Injury	Victim impacted against stationary object
Quaternary Blast Injury	Burns, inhalation injuries, crush injuries

Mechanisms of Blast Injuries

Prognostic factors which affect the mortality and morbidity of blast injuries include:

- Victim orientation to the blast
- Magnitude of the blast
- Environment of the blast (outdoor vs. indoor vs. underwater)
- Structural collapse
- Triage accuracy
- Available medical resources.

KEY POINTS

 The effects of a blast are increased in a "closed" space such as a building or a bus.

 Quaternary injuries resulting from blasts include crush injuries, thermal injuries, and compartment syndrome.

 Most survivors of blast injuries sustain mixed types of blast injury.

 Blast injury + building collapse is associated with the highest mortality and morbidity.

147

Crush Injuries

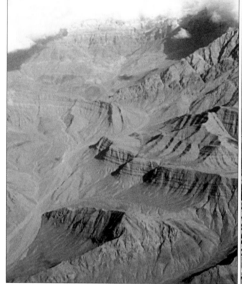 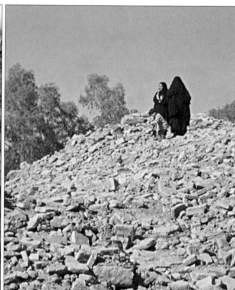

Figs. 14.1, 14.2 Iran earthquake (2003)

CASE SCENARIO

A magnitude 6.6 earthquake struck Bam, Iran at 5:26 AM on December 26, 2003 while most people were asleep in their beds. Bam is situated between the Jebal Barez Mountains and the Lut Desert at 1,060 meters above sea level in southeastern Iran. The human and physical devastation was staggering with over 41,000 victims killed and tens of thousands injured. Nearly all the survivors were homeless. A request for international disaster relief was made by Iran. Twenty-four search and rescue teams and 13 field hospitals, including a team from the United States, responded to the request.

Introduction

Crush injury is defined as compression of extremities and body parts that causes muscle swelling and/or neurological disturbances in the affected parts of the body. Typically affected body parts include lower extremities (74%), upper extremities (10%), and trunk (9%).

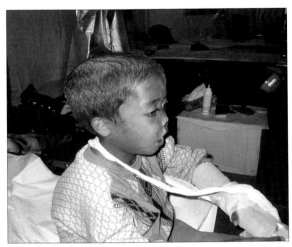

Fig. 14.3 Crush injury victim,
Pakistan earthquake, (2005)

Crush syndrome is localized crush injury with systemic manifestations. These systemic effects are caused by a *traumatic rhabdomyolysis* (muscle breakdown) and the release of potentially toxic muscle cell components and electrolytes into the circulation.

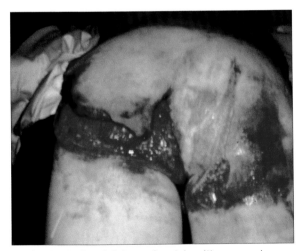

Fig. 14.4 Crush injury of pelvis with secondary crush syndrome.

Crush Injury

Crush injury is the compression of extremities and body parts causing localized muscle and nerve damage. Crush injuries often occur after bombings, industrial accidents, building collapse, earthquakes, and tornadoes.

Crush Syndrome

Crush syndrome can cause local tissue injury, organ dysfunction, and metabolic abnormalities such as acidosis (low blood pH levels), *hyperkalemia* (high potassium levels), and *hypocalcemia* (low calcium levels).

Previous experience with earthquakes that caused major structural damage demonstrated that:

- The incidence of crush syndrome was 2-15%.

- Approximately half of those with crush syndrome developed acute renal failure.

- Approximately half of those with acute renal failure needed dialysis.

- A significant number of patients (>50%) with crush syndrome needed fasciotomy.

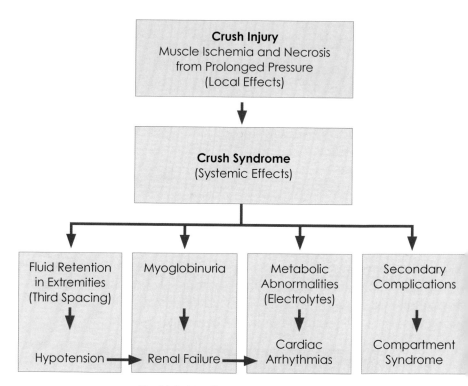

Fig.14.5 Manifestations of crush injury

Clinical Manifestations of Crush Syndrome

Sudden release of a crushed extremity may result in acute hypovolemia and metabolic abnormalities (reperfusion syndrome). This may cause lethal cardiac arrhythmias and sudden death. Further, the sudden release of toxins from necrotic muscle into the circulation leads to *myoglobinuria* (excretion of myoglobin in the urine), which causes renal failure if untreated.

Hypotension

Massive third spacing occurs, requiring massive fluid replacement in the first 24 hours.

- Shock may contribute to renal failure.

- Third spacing may lead to secondary complications such as *compartment syndrome* (swelling within a closed anatomical space).

Renal Failure

- Rhabdomyolysis releases myoglobin, potassium, phosphorous, and creatinine into circulation.

- Myoglobinuria may result in renal tubular necrosis.

- Release of electrolytes from ischemic muscle causes metabolic abnormalities.

Metabolic Abnormalities

- Calcium flows into muscle cells through leaky membranes, causing systemic hypocalcemia.

- Potassium is released from ischemic muscle into systemic circulation, causing hyperkalemia.

- Lactic acid is released from ischemic muscle into systemic circulation, causing metabolic acidosis.

- Imbalance of potassium and calcium may cause life-threatening cardiac arrhythmias, including cardiac arrest. Metabolic acidosis may exacerbate this situation.

Secondary Complications

- Compartment syndrome may occur, which will further worsen vascular compromise.

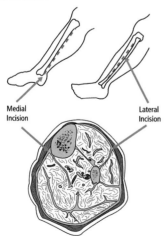

Fig. 14.6 Four-compartment fasciotomy using two-incision technique.

151

Definitive Management of Crush Syndrome

- Pretreat casualties with intravenous (IV) fluids before release of crushing object whenever possible. If this is not possible, consider applying a tourniquet to the affected limb.

- Field amputation of a crushed extremity is considered as a last resort for extrication of a critically ill patient.

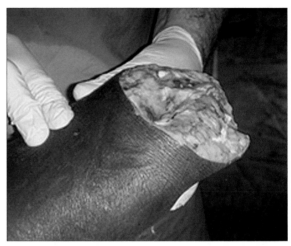

Fig. 14.7 Field amputation, Haiti earthquake (2010)

Hypotension
Crush syndrome can cause massive fluid shifts in casualties.
- Initiate (or continue) IV hydration—1 to 1.5 L/hour.

- Patients may gain up to 20-50 pounds in fluid weight.

Renal Failure
- If available, use urine dipsticks to check for myoglobin to detect patients at risk for subclinical myoglobinuria. If the urine is dark, assume myoglobinuria and an increased risk for renal failure.

- Prevent renal failure through appropriate hydration.

- Maintain diuresis of 300 cc/hr with IV fluids and mannitol.

  o Initial resuscitation with Normal Saline (may require over 1-1.5 L/hour to maintain urine output).

  o To alkalinize urine, add 2 amps (100mEq) sodium bicarbonate to 1 liter D5W and administer as continuous infusion. Titrate to urine pH >6.5.

  o Administration of mannitol may be considered once urine flow is established (20% mannitol, 1-2gm/kg every 4 hrs as needed, not to exceed 200g/day).

TREATMENT ALERT!

Pretreat casualties with prolonged crush (>4 hours), as well as those who demonstrate an abnormal neurological or vascular exam, with 1-2 liters of Normal Saline before releasing crushing object whenever possible.

If not possible, apply tourniquets to crushed limbs and maintain until initiation of IV fluids.

- Triage to hemodialysis as needed.
    - o Each patient may need up to 60 days' treatment.
    - o Unless sepsis is present, renal failure may completely resolve with treatment.
    - o Highest priority for dialysis should be for patients with oliguric renal failure and those with severe hyperkalemia not responsive to medical therapy.

Metabolic Abnormalities

- **Acidosis:** Administer IV sodium bicarbonate until urine pH reaches 6.5 to prevent myoglobin deposition in kidneys.
- **Hyperkalemia/Hypocalcemia:** Administer calcium, sodium bicarbonate, and insulin/glucose; consider Kayexalate.
- **Cardiac Arrhythmias:** Electrolyte imbalances can cause life-threatening cardiac arrhythmias, including cardiac arrest. Monitor for cardiac arrhythmias and treat accordingly.

Secondary Complications

- Monitor casualties for symptoms of compartment syndrome, including pain, pallor, paresthesias, pain with passive movement, and pulselessness. Monitor compartment pressures if equipment is available. If compartment syndrome occurs, consider emergency fasciotomy.
- Late fasciotomy, more than 12 hours after development of compartment syndrome, is controversial due to concern for increased risk of infection without further limb-salvage advantage.

> **TREATMENT ALERT!**
>
> Monitor for vascular compromise/compartment syndrome using the five P's:
> - Pain
> - Pallor
> - Paresthesias
> - Pain with passive movement
> - Pulselessness

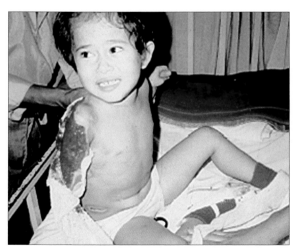

Fig. 14.8 Crush injury victim, El Salvador earthquake (1987).

- Treat open wounds with debridement of necrotic tissue, tetanus toxoid, and antibiotics if wound is infected. **Note that infected wounds in an earthquake setting will often be polymicrobial infections with atypical bacteria and thus require administration of broad-spectrum antibiotics.**

- Apply ice to injured areas.

- Delays of hydration for longer than 12 hours increase the incidence of renal failure.

- Overall mortality for acute renal failure in an earthquake setting ranges from 14-48%. Most common cause of mortality after crush injury is sepsis.

Summary

Crush injuries are common in both natural and man-made disasters, especially if complicated by building collapse. Aggressive, early treatment of crush injury victims is the key to reducing mortality and morbidity and the incidence of secondary complications such as crush syndrome.

KEY POINTS

 Crush injury is defined as compression of extremities and body parts that causes muscle swelling and/or neurological disturbances in the affected parts of the body.

 Crush syndrome is localized crush injury with systemic manifestations.

 Pretreat crush casualties with intravenous Normal Saline **before** releasing crushing object whenever possible.

 Monitor victims of crush injury for metabolic abnormalities and compartment syndrome.

Pediatric Disaster Response:
Resuscitation, Trauma, and Critical Illnesses

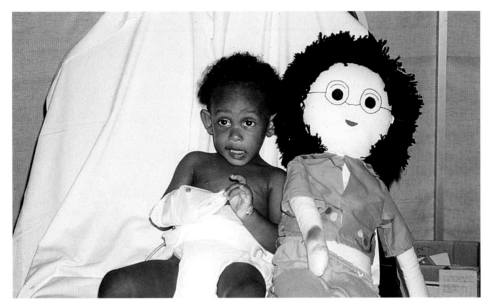

Figure 15.1 Child with Ciguatera (fish) poisioning, Hurricane Marilyn (1995)

CASE SCENARIO

Hurricane Marilyn struck the US Virgin Islands on September 15-16, 1995, with sustained winds of over 110 mph. The only hospital was badly damaged, including the entire pediatric ward, which was the regional center for neonatal and pediatric care. Disaster teams with pediatric expertise were deployed from the USA to assist in the care of the victims. Children were disproportionately impacted by the disaster, presenting with traumatic injuries and exacerbation of pre-existing diseases such as asthma and critical illnesses.

Introduction

Most disasters involve significant numbers of children as well as adults. Differences in injury patterns, illnesses, anatomy, physiology, and psychosocial development in children require age-specific evaluation and management for successful care of pediatric disaster victims. It is critical to develop a comprehensive plan for preparation and response that addresses initial stabilization and definitive care of injuries and illnesses.

Preparation for pediatric disaster response begins long before a disaster occurs. Disaster medical teams should include healthcare providers trained in the care of children with critical injuries and illnesses. This may include those who specialize in pediatric emergency medicine, general surgery, orthopedics, anesthesia, and other pediatric sub-specialties. Pediatric staffing requirements are based on the number of children expected to be seen each day, with a ratio of approximately five registered nurses and two pediatric-trained physicians to treat 100 children.

Preparation for Disasters

Pediatric Equipment
Commonly used equipment:

- Cardiorespiratory monitor
- Nebulizer
- Pulse oximeter

Pediatric Supplies
Commonly used supplies:

- Wound care supplies
- Dressings
- Face masks, nasal cannulas
- Intraosseous (IO) needles (preferably with an automated device)
- Intravenous (IV) catheterization supplies (20, 22, 24 gauge catheters)
- Nasogastric, orogastric tubes ≥ 8 French (Fr), suction canisters
- Neonatal resuscitation supplies
- Otoscope/ophthalmoscope/ear specula
- Spacer devices for metered dose inhalers
- Suction catheters (≥ 6 Fr)
- Suturing supplies
- Urinary catheters (≥ 6 Fr)

Uncommonly used supplies:

- Defibrillator/automated external defibrillator (AED)
- Capnography
- Chest tubes ≥ 10 Fr, pleurovac
- Cervical spine collars
- Intubation supplies:
  - o Endotracheal tubes (ETT) with stylets (cuffed ≥ 3.0 Fr) (uncuffed 2.5-3.5 Fr)
  - o Laryngoscope/blades (Miller 0, 1, 2, 3) (Macintosh or Wis-Hipple 2, 3)
- Nasopharyngeal, oral airways

Desirable equipment:

- Ultrasound
- Video-assisted laryngoscope

Pediatric Fluids

Commonly used fluids:

- Normal Saline
- Lactated Ringer's
- D5 1/2 Normal Saline

Uncommonly used fluids:

- Blood products

Pediatric Drugs

Commonly used drugs:

- Acyclovir
- Antibiotics
- Antipyretics
- Analgesics
- Bronchodilators
- Corticosteroids
- IV/oral rehydration solutions
- Local anesthetics
- Sedatives (minor)
- Vaccines

Uncommonly used drugs:

- Anticonvulsants
- Diuretics
- Glucose

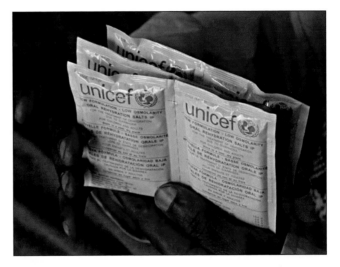

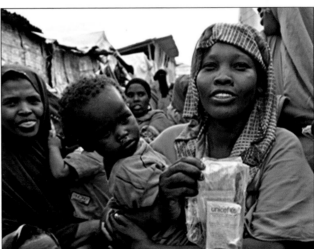

Figs. 15.2, 15.3 Oral rehydration solutions, Courtesy of UNICEF

- Major sedatives
- Resuscitation (Pediatric Advanced Life Support) medications
- Neonatal resuscitation (Neonatal Acute Life Support) medications

Rarely used drugs:

- Antidotes
- Antihypertensives
- Antipsychotics
- Insulin

Triage and Assessment

Initial triage of pediatric disaster victims is performed using the same triage principles as for adults, but with different parameters. Both pediatric triage and assessment require knowledge of age-appropriate vital signs, physical exam findings, mental status, cognitive development, and motor skills.

Pediatric triage and assessment are crucial skills that should be a core focus of disaster-training programs. It requires a knowledge of the injuries and illnesses to which children are most vulnerable as a result of disasters. In pediatric patients, initial presentation may not reflect severity of injury or illness, and their condition may deteriorate quickly. It is not always obvious, particularly for providers with limited pediatric experience, that a child is in, or on the precipice of, distress or extremis. Frequent reassessment, anticipation and proactive interventions are essential to reverse and ideally prevent deterioration.

PEDIATRIC VITAL SIGNS: NORMAL VALUES

Age	Heart Rate (beats/min)	Respiratory Rate (breaths/min)
Infant	100-160	30-60
Toddler	90-150	24-40
Preschooler	80-140	22-34
School-age	70-120	18-30
Adolescent	60-100	12-16

Pediatric Resuscitation

Resuscitation in pediatric patients is made more challenging by the requirement for age-or weight-based equipment, supplies, and medications. **Dosing tapes, such as the Broselow-Luten tape, provide equipment sizes and medication doses based on patient length as a proxy for weight.** The Broselow-Luten tape is particularly helpful when age is not known, as is common in disaster settings. However, it is important to note that tapes based on US pediatric norms for height and weight may not be applicable in international deployments, requiring healthcare providers to adjust the results. Tables with similar information and several mobile applications that calculate appropriate sizes and doses based on age and/or weight can also be used to provide this information.

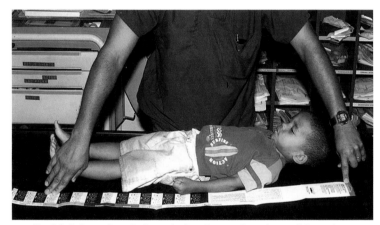

Fig.15.4 Broselow-Luten dosing tape, Courtesy of Broselow

Principles of resuscitation are similar to that of adults; however, causes of cardiopulmonary compromise/arrest differ. **Unlike adults, in children 95% of cardiac arrests are the result of respiratory compromise.** Early recognition and aggressive management of respiratory compromise are critical to prevent life-threatening decompensation. The prognosis for pediatric arrest, particularly outside of the healthcare environment, is exceedingly poor. This reality must be considered when allocating scarce human and physical resources during a disaster. Tachypnea is an early sign of respiratory distress and may be followed by flaring, retractions, and/or grunting. **Bradypnea is a late finding and an ominous sign for impending respiratory arrest followed by cardiopulmonary arrest.**

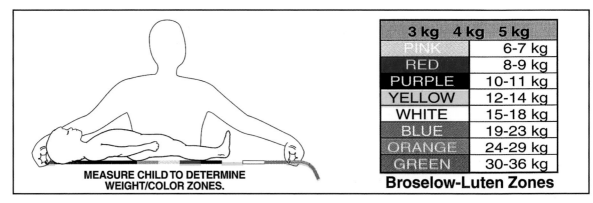

3 kg	**4 kg**	**5 kg**	
PINK			6-7 kg
RED			8-9 kg
PURPLE			10-11 kg
YELLOW			12-14 kg
WHITE			15-18 kg
BLUE			19-23 kg
ORANGE			24-29 kg
GREEN			30-36 kg

MEASURE CHILD TO DETERMINE WEIGHT/COLOR ZONES.

Broselow-Luten Zones

Fig.15.5 Broselow-Luten dosing tape, Courtesy of Broselow

Airway

Proper positioning of the patient to achieve maximum airway patency must take into account that the disproportionately large occiput of small children places their neck in flexion, causing buckling of the airway.

- **To attain anatomic sniffing position, a roll under the shoulder blades may be required.**

- Chin lift (or jaw thrust in children with potential c-spine injury) should be performed to open the airway, with recognition that the relatively large tongue may occlude the airway and may need to be repositioned.

Oral secretions, blood clots, teeth, or other foreign bodies or debris may also obstruct the narrow pediatric airway. Oral suctioning may be required, but should be performed cautiously to avoid further obstructing the airway. **Infants < 4 months of age are obligate nose breathers, so nasal obstruction can cause significant respiratory distress.** A nasal airway, or an oral airway in an unresponsive child, may serve as an adjunct to establish and maintain airway patency. In children, unlike in adults, an oral airway should be inserted with the outer portion of the curve toward the palate to prevent soft-tissue injury to the palate.

For the child with insufficient or absent respiratory effort and/or airway narrowing that compromises ventilatory function, bag-valve mask ventilation should be initiated while preparing for intubation. The appropriate size mask is one that fits over the bridge of the nose and in the cleft of the chin.

Pre-oxygenation prior to intubation is particularly important in children because of their relatively limited respiratory reserve. **Oxygen should be delivered for 3-5 minutes prior to attempting intubation.** Oropharyngeal intubation is preferred to nasopharyngeal intubation in pediatric patients because their more anterior larynx and more anterocaudally angled vocal cords make nasopharyngeal intubation quite difficult.

Endotracheal tube selection is age-based. **Cuffed tubes are preferred for patients beyond the neonatal period.**

- As with adults, if airway edema is present, the size of the ETT tube will need to be reduced.

- The depth of the ETT is usually approximately three times the internal diameter of the tube, as calculated for an uncuffed tube, (e.g., a 3.0 Fr tube is inserted to approximately 9 cm at the lip). Listening for breath sounds at the anterior axillary line bilaterally helps to assure that breath sounds heard on one side are not transmitted from the other side.

- The child's trachea is much shorter than that of an adult. Right-sided intubation is more common than left given the straighter right mainstem bronchus. Direct visualization, symmetric chest rise and breath sounds, and end-tidal CO_2 should be used as indicators of appropriate tube placement.

- While chest x-ray provides definitive confirmation of ETT placement, radiology is usually not practical, given limited availability and the resources required for transport of unstable patients to x-ray.

- **A laryngeal mask airway (LMA) is an acceptable short-term option if an ETT is not available or cannot be placed. For providers with limited pediatric intubation experience, LMA placement may be associated with fewer complications than ETT placement.**

Etomidate for induction and the nondepolarizing neuromuscular blockers, rocuronium or vecuronium for paralysis, are appropriate agents for rapid-sequence intubation in the conscious patient.

- Lidocaine can be considered in patients with concern for increased intracranial pressure.

- Atropine can be considered in infants < 1 year of age to prevent bradycardia during intubation, but current literature does not compellingly support its use.

- Benzodiazepines and opiates should be administered as needed to maintain sedation in the intubated patient.

- Succinylcholine can be considered in patients with presumed difficult airways, provided no contraindications to the drug exist.

TREATMENT ALERT!

Tube size can be calculated based on age for children 1-10 years:

- Cuffed tube size (mm ID) = (age in years/4) + 3

- Uncuffed tube size (mm ID) = (age in years/4) + 4

RISK ALERT!

Flexion or extension of the child's neck may be enough to displace the endotracheal tube. Secure endotracheal tubes in place with umbilical or tracheal tape rather than adhesive tape when possible.

Breathing

Signs of respiratory distress in children include tachypnea, nasal flaring, retractions, and grunting. Patients with respiratory compromise or potential for compromise should be monitored by pulse oximetry. Pediatric patients are often the first to display respiratory manifestations resulting from exposure to dust, smoke, and other environmental particulate matter, as well as biological, chemical, and radioactive agents. Even in neonates and infants, bronchodilators can be administered by an inhaler with a spacer.

- **Oxygen should be provided at the concentration necessary to maintain saturations at 100% during resuscitation and > 94% once the child has been stabilized.**

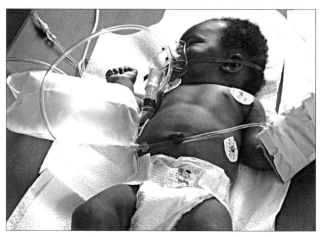

Fig.15.6 Child with respiratory distress, Haiti earthquake (2010)

- Patients requiring supplemental oxygen should ideally be monitored by capnography using inline end-tidal CO_2.

- Breaths delivered should not exceed the minimum volume and force required to produce chest rise. Risks of over-ventilation include impeding venous return, air trapping, gastric distension, regurgitation, and aspiration.

- A nasogastric or orogastric tube should be placed to prevent/ decompress abdominal distension, which can restrict lung expansion, especially in young children.

Circulation

- Children, particularly neonates and infants, become dehydrated more quickly than adults, yet they have remarkable cardiovascular reserve. Tachycardia is an indicator of moderate to severe dehydration and one of the first indicators of shock. **Hypotension is a late finding of shock, not seen until at least 20-25% of fluid and/or blood volume is lost.**

Initial fluid resuscitation with Normal Saline or Ringer's Lactate, 10 mL/kg for neonates and 20 mL/kg for infants and children, is recommended. If hemodynamic status has not been restored with 40-60 mL/kg crystalloid, pressors and/or if there has been significant blood loss, packed red blood cells (PRBC's) should be administered. Two large-bore IVs should be placed in all critically-injured or ill children with circulatory compromise.

Options for venous access:

- Peripheral veins

  o Preferred sites are antecubital, saphenous, hand and foot veins. Scalp vein may be an option in infants.

  o Umbilical vein may be an option in neonates during the first week of life.

- IO infusion

If attempts at peripheral access fail, an intraosseous needle should be placed. Do not delay IO placement in a child in extremis when IV attempts are unsuccessful. Preferred intraosseous site is the anteromedial tibia 1-3 cm inferior to the growth plate, directed away from the growth plate. If lower legs are injured or tibial IO placement/function has failed, IO should be placed into the anterior midline femur, 1-3 cm proximal to the superior aspect of the patella directed away from the growth plate. **All drugs that can be administered IV can be administered via intraosseous infusion.**

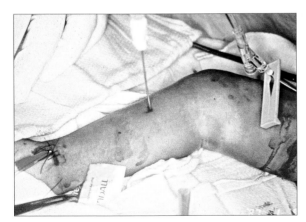

Fig. 15.7 Intraosseous fluid resuscitation

- Central vein access

  o The preferred site for central lines, particularly in young children, is the femoral vein, followed by the internal jugular vein.

163

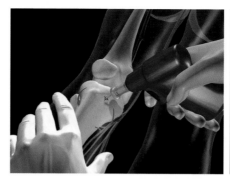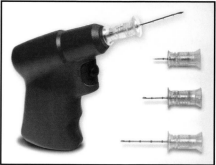

Figs. 15.8, 15.9 EZ-IO Intraosseus Infusion System, Courtesy of VIDACARE

Cardiac Dysfunction

The most common pediatric arrhythmias are disturbances of rate, i.e., bradycardia, tachycardia and supraventricular tachycardia. Rhythm disturbances include asystole, pulseless electrical activity, pulseless ventricular tachycardia (VT) and ventricular fibrillation (VF).

Asystole

- **The outcome for children presenting in asystole from an out-of-hospital arrest is very poor.** Rapid intervention may improve the chances of successful resuscitation.

- As of 2010, guidelines for initial management include immediate initiation of chest compressions and subsequent assessment of the airway and provision of adequate ventilation. Compressions of at least one-third the diameter of the chest, 4 cm (1.5 in) for infants and 5 cm (2 in) for children, at a rate of at least 100 per minute should be delivered with the child laying on a hard surface.

- Drug of choice in asystole is epinephrine given via IV/IO, or if access cannot be achieved, endotracheally. IV/IO administration is dosed at 0.1 mL/kg of a **1:10,000** solution (equivalent to 0.01 mg/kg).

- For children, the ratio of compressions to breaths is 15:2 with two rescuers. At the age of puberty, this changes to the adult ratio of 30:2.

- If the endotracheal route must be utilized, the **1:1,000** concentration is dosed at 0.1 mL/kg (equivalent to 0.1 mg/kg). To ensure adequate dispersal in the lungs, installation should be followed by 3 to 5 mL of Normal Saline and five positive-pressure breaths. Epinephrine doses are repeated every 3 to 5 minutes. Vasopressin, used to treat cardiac arrests in adults, does not have a role in pediatric cardiac arrests at present due to a lack of data to support its use.

Pulseless Electrical Activity (PEA)

PEA is characterized by cardiac activity without central pulses. Reversible causes of PEA are referred to as the H's and T's.

REVERSIBLE CAUSES OF PEA: H'S AND T'S

Hypoxia	Tamponade
Hypothermia	Tension pneumothorax
Hypovolemia	Toxins
Hydrogen ion (acidosis)	Trauma
Hypo/Hyperkalemia	Thromboembolism

Advanced Cardiac Life Support, American Heart Association (AHA)

If any of these conditions exist, it is essential to recognize and correct them immediately. The drug of choice for PEA is epinephrine, dosed as above for asystole.

Pulseless Ventricular Tachycardia (VT) and Ventricular Fibrillation (VF)

Initial treatment for pulseless VT or VF is defibrillation.

- Compressions should be initiated as soon as the patient is determined to be pulseless and continued until AED/defibrillator is available.

- An AED that has pediatric pads or a converter cable should be used in children who have not reached puberty. However, if the only available AED is configured for adults, it should still be used. The use of adult pads on an infant may require front and back placement.

- In the treatment of pulseless VT or VF, a single "shock" is given with immediate resumption of cardiopulmonary resuscitation (CPR). Following subsequent shocks, circulation is reassessed.

- **The vast majority of defibrillators manufactured today are biphasic. The initial energy settings for children are weight-based starting at 2 to 4 joules/kg, with subsequent energy levels of at least 4 joules/kg, not to exceed 10 joules/kg.**

- For adolescents and adults, initial energy level should be 150 joules, and increased to 200 joules for subsequent shocks.

- If an older monophasic defibrillator is used, the initial settings for children are the same weight based 2-10 joules/kg.

Concurrent treatment of pulseless VT or VF includes epinephrine.
Each dose of medication given in VF/pulseless VT should be followed by a defibrillating shock. If no response is seen following the initial two doses of epinephrine, an antiarrhythmic medication, either amiodarone or lidocaine is inidicated.

Amiodarone slows conduction through the atrioventricular node secondary to the delay in repolarization. Amiodarone is dosed at 5 mg/kg (maximum 300 mg/dose) given as a rapid IV/IO bolus. In stable VT, amiodarone is further diluted in 10 to 20 mL of NS or D5W and infused over 20 to 60 minutes. Amiodarone has an extended half-life, and it is important to note that significant drug-drug interactions can occur days to weeks after initial administration.

Adverse effects are common and can include complete heart block, hypotension, and arrhythmias. **Amiodarone should not be given concurrently with procainamide or other class I antiarrhythmic agents due to prolongation of the QTc interval.**

Lidocaine is a class 1b antiarrhythmic agent that suppresses the automaticity of ventricles and the His-Purkinje system. Lidocaine is dosed at 1 to 1.5 mg/kg via IV/IO as a rapid bolus. The dose can be repeated at 50% of the original dose (0.5 to 0.75 mg/kg) every 3 to 5 minutes until a maximum of 3 mg/kg is reached. It is important to highlight that there is no evidence supporting amiodarone as superior to lidocaine in pediatric VF/pulseless VT.

In torsades de pointes, the drug of choice is magnesium sulfate 25 to 50 mg/kg (max 2,000 mg/dose), diluted and run over 10 to 20 minutes.

Bradycardia
Early correction of underlying causes such as hypoxia and hypothermia is essential. The first-line medication for bradycardia in children is epinephrine. Atropine is no longer recommended as a primary drug for children and should be used only when a vagal cause is suspected. Atropine is dosed at 0.02 mg/kg (minimum dose 0.1 mg, maximum dose 1 mg) given IV/IO. It is important to note that atropine's mydriatic effects on the pupils may last several hours, making pupillary (and thus the neurological) exam more difficult to interpret. Cardiac pacing may be necessary to maintain perfusion for patients in a bradycardic rhythm.

TREATMENT ALERT!

Atropine is used in treatment of bradycardia only when a vagal cause is suspected.

Supraventricular Tachycardia

Supraventricular tachycardia (SVT) is distinguished from sinus tachycardia by a heart rate that is >220 beats per minute (bpm) in children < 1 year of age and 180 bpm in children > 1 year old. In SVT, heart rate is constant without beat-to-beat variability, p-waves are absent and QRS waves are narrow complex. An important distinction when assessing the patient for therapy is the presence of poor perfusion and/or hypotension. If either one or both are present, the patient is considered to be unstable and should be immediately cardioverted.

Cardioversion is synchronized, and the energy should initially be set at 0.5-1 joules/kg (max 100 joules) and increased to 2 joules/kg (max 200 joules) for subsequent shocks. As with defibrillation, the energy settings may vary between monophasic and biphasic machines, so it is important to become familiar with the available equipment. When time allows, sedation and analgesia with agents such as midazolam and fentanyl are recommended, as synchronized cardioversion can be extremely unpleasant. In the stable patient, vagal maneuvers should be employed initially while access is obtained. These include placing ice on the face and/or having the patient blow through an occluded straw or bear down as if having a bowel movement.

The first-line pharmacologic agent for the treatment of SVT is adenosine. Due to the ultra-short half-life of adenosine in vivo, all doses should be given as centrally as possible, although peripheral vein and IO administration are acceptable. Administration should be immediately followed by a saline flush. A three-way stopcock is often used to facilitate this process. The dose of adenosine is 0.1 mg/kg (max 6 mg) via rapid IV push for the first dose, followed by 0.2 mg/kg (max 12 mg) via rapid IV push if the initial dose was unsuccessful at converting the patient to normal sinus rhythm. A short period of asystole when conduction is interrupted via the atrioventricular (AV) node allows the heart to resume normal sinus rhythm.

Procainamide is used as a second-line drug when adenosine is not successful. The dose of procainamide is 15 mg/kg administered over 30 to 60 minutes. Adverse effects requiring immediate interruption of infusion include hypotension and prolongation of the QT interval. Continuous infusion of procainamide may also be necessary to control the arrhythmia. Other alternatives for converting SVT may include beta-blockers, verapamil (not for children < 1 year of age), and digoxin.

Pediatric Arrhythmias

Arrhythmia	Intervention	Dose	Comments
Asystole	Epinephrine 1:10,000	0.01 mg/kg (0.1 mL/kg)	Repeat every 3-5 minutes
Pulseless VT/VF	Defibrillation	2-4 joules/kg, increase up to 10 joules/kg	
	Epinephrine 1:10,000	0.01 mg/kg (0.1 mL/kg)	Repeat every 3-5 minutes
	Amiodarone	5 mg/kg	Maximum 300 mg/dose
	Lidocaine	1 mg/kg	Maximum 100 mg/dose
PEA	Epinephrine 1:10,000	0.01 mg/kg (0.1 mL/kg)	Repeat every 3-5 minutes
Bradycardia	Epinephrine 1:10,000	0.01 mg/kg (0.1 mL/kg)	Repeat every 3-5 minutes
	Pacing (Set desired rate and set output beginning with 30 mA, increase until capture.)		
SVT	Adenosine	Initial dose: 0.1 mg/kg	Initial dose: maximum 6 mg/dose
	Synchronized cardioversion	0.5-2 joules/kg	Sedate prior if no hypotension. Do not delay if hypotension present.
	Procainamide (Over 30-45 minutes)	• Age < 1 year 7-10 mg/kg • > 1 year 15 mg/kg	
Torsades de pointes	Magnesium sulfate	25-50 mg/kg	Maximum 2,000 mg/dose

Specific Patterns of Injury in Children

Neurological Injuries

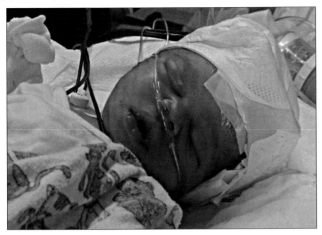

Fig. 15.10 Child with crush injury to head,
Haiti earthquake (2010)

Head injuries alone or associated with other injuries are responsible for most of the fatal traumatic injuries in children. The disproportionately large head size of young children increases their risk of head injury. The smaller brain-to-cranium size and weaker neck musculature increases their risk of acceleration/deceleration injury. Greater blood flow to the brain in children increases their risk of cerebral edema from hypoxia, hypovolemia, and hyperthermia. Brain plasticity allows for better long-term outcome in children than in adults.

The Glasgow Coma Score for children can be used as a guide to severity of injury, which directly correlates with outcome:

- 13-15 = mild
- 9-12 = moderate
- 5-8 = severe
- 3-4 = very severe

Glasgow Coma Score for Children

Eye Opening (E)	Verbal Response (V) < 4 years of age	Verbal Response (V) 4+ years of age	Motor Response (M)
4=Spontaneous 3=To voice 2=To pain 1=None	5=Appropriate words or social smiles, fixes on objects/voice 4=Cries, but consolable 3=Persistently irritable 2=Restless, agitated 1=None	5=Normal conversation 4=Disoriented conversation 3=Words, but not coherent 2=No words: only sounds 1=None	6=Normal 5=Localizes to pain 4=Withdraws to pain 3=Decorticate posture 2=Decerebrate 1=None
TOTAL = E+V+M			

Pediatric patients who have suffered an isolated head injury, even if alert and awake at the time of examination, should be triaged to hospital care if they exhibit any one of the following:

- Loss of consciousness
- Altered level of consciousness, sleepiness, confusion and/or agitation
- Seizures
- Focal neurologic deficit
- Evidence of a cerebrospinal fluid (CSF) leak
- Persistent vomiting

Cervical Spine Injuries

Traumatic spinal cord injuries are uncommon in children, particularly neonates and infants, even if they have sustained head trauma. For children with more than minor injury and/or decreased conciousness following injury, strict precautions are necessary until a cervical spine injury is ruled out. In young children, approximate age < 5 years, the c-spine usually cannot be reliably cleared clinically. When available, x-ray is preferable to computed tomography (CT) to clear the pediatric c-spine.

Children > 15 years of age generally have adult patterns of spinal cord injuries and can undergo an evaluation similar to that of an adult. **However, children under 8 years of age are particularly susceptible to SCIWORA (spinal cord injury without radiographic abnormality).** The immature and relatively lax cervical ligaments, incomplete bone ossification, and horizontally oriented articular surfaces of the vertebral bodies in children put young patients at higher risk for subluxation and spinal cord injury. In addition, the relatively larger head and immature neck musculature in children leads to a fulcrum effect in the C1 to C3 area. Younger children, therefore, often suffer a higher level of cervical spine injury than adults.

Subluxation of C2 on C3 is a normal variant in 40% of children < 7 years old and 20% < 14 years old. Patients with unstable c-spine fractures will require c-spine stabilization. Those with stable fractures, SCIWORA, or c-spine tenderness without obvious fracture should remain in a hard collar with close follow-up.

Thoracic Injuries

Thoracic injury is the second most common cause of mortality in the pediatric trauma patient. Greater than two-thirds of patients with thoracic injury have other organ-system injuries. The majority of thoracic injuries in children are secondary to blunt force, although the incidence of penetrating trauma to the chest is increased in adolescents. Anatomic features particular to children make the injury patterns and treatments different.

Rib Fractures

Children have much more compliant chest walls. Rib fractures, therefore, are much less common, and severe thoracic injuries may occur without significant external evidence of trauma.

When rib fractures are present, it is likely an indicator of more severe underlying injury. There should be careful monitoring, a low threshold for further testing, if available, and aggressive management of respiratory distress. Treatment of rib fractures involves pain control and rest. Most rib fractures heal within six weeks.

Pulmonary Contusion

Pulmonary contusion is one of the most common injuries in blunt thoracic trauma in the pediatric population. Although patients may have overlying abrasions, contusions, or rib fractures, the injury may not be clinically apparent. Pulmonary contusion is not always seen on chest x-ray. CT is more sensitive. However, imaging specifically for pulmonary contusion is usually not necessary, because treatment is support of ventilation, as clinically required.

Pneumothorax and Hemothorax

Asymmetric chest rise and/or breath sounds may indicate pneumothorax or hemothorax and may be appreciated before the onset of respiratory distress.

- Mediastinal structures are more mobile in children than in adults.

- Tension pneumothorax, caused by a shift of mediastinal structures, may result in life-threatening cardiorespiratory compromise.

- Tension pneumothorax should always be considered as a possible diagnosis in the hypotensive, hypoxic patient.

- Management of pneumothorax and hemothorax is similar in adults and children. In general, chest tube placement at the level of the nipple (approximately fourth or fifth intercostal space) in the midaxillary line is appropriate.

- **For tension pneumothorax, needle decompression at the second intercostal space followed by chest tube placement is life-saving and must be performed swiftly.**

RECOMMENDED CHEST TUBE SIZES

- Newborns - 12 to 16 Fr
- Infants - 16 to 18 Fr
- Younger children - 18 to 24 Fr
- Adolescents - 28 to 32 Fr

Traumatic Asphyxia

Traumatic asphyxia is an injury seen almost exclusively in children. This occurs with sudden compression of the abdomen and/or chest against a closed glottis. There is a rapid rise in intrathoracic pressure, which is transmitted to all of the veins that drain into the valveless superior vena cava. Capillary extravasation occurs in the upper half of the body, sclerae, and sometimes the brain.

Signs and symptoms include:

- Hyperemic sclera
- Seizures
- Disorientation
- Petechiae in the upper half of the body
- Respiratory failure

Traumatic asphyxia is a clinical diagnosis and has a good prognosis. Treatment is supportive. Associated injuries include pulmonary contusions, central nervous system (CNS) injuries, and intra-abdominal injuries.

Abdominal Injuries

Abdominal injury in children is likely to result from blunt trauma. Spleen, liver, and kidney are the most commonly injured, followed by the intestine, pancreas, and urinary bladder. Isolated abdominal injuries account for approximately 10% of childhood trauma-related deaths, while 70% of fatalities result from severe head injuries associated with abdominal injuries.

Children are more prone to abdominal injuries than adults because their rib cages are smaller and more pliable, therefore offering less protection to the upper abdominal viscera. **Children's organs are relatively larger in relation to the abdomen, making them more vulnerable to injury.** Moreover, the thin abdominal wall musculature provides less protection from both blunt and penetrating trauma. Serial examinations are essential as young children are often not able to provide a full history or cooperate with the initial examination.

Ultrasound FAST exam to diagnose intra-abdominal trauma is not as sensitive in children as in adults. The diagnosis is based on the presence of intra-abdominal free fluid, which is less likely to be present in children due to more distensible solid organ capsules.

Splenic Injuries
The spleen is the most commonly injured abdominal organ in children. The vast majority of splenic injuries can be managed non-operatively. Non-operative management is particularly important to children, as they are at increased risk for post-splenectomy bacterial sepsis.

Hepatic Injuries
The liver is the second-most commonly injured organ in the child's abdomen. **The majority of hepatic injuries can be managed non-operatively.**

Kidney Injuries
Injury to the kidney may result not only in bleeding but also extravasation of urine and/or compromised renal function. Most renal injuries can be managed non-operatively.

Duodenal and Stomach Injuries
Intramural duodenal hematoma is the most common small bowel injury in children. It occurs as the duodenum is forced posteriorly against the vertebral body. Symptoms include post-prandial epigastric and right-upper quadrant pain occurring immediately to seven days following the initial injury. Persistent bilious emesis is common. Stomach rupture is rare, but can occur following an abrupt blunt force to the abdomen following a full meal.

Orthopedic Injuries
In the patient with multiple trauma, orthopedic injuries often coexist with other injuries. Although sometimes difficult, it is essential to obtain a thorough history and careful neurovascular examination.

The major differences between adults' and childrens' bones are:

- Presence of the *physis*, e.g., "growth plate"
- Lesser bone density
- Greater plasticity and greater capacity for remodeling

These differences result in fractures that are unique to children. Fractures in children heal more rapidly with greater capacity to restore anatomic alignment and lower risk of non-union. **It is essential to provide proper traction and splinting to prevent further soft tissue damage and pain for the patient prior to further trauma evaluation.** Length of immobilization depends on the age of the child and the forces specific to the bone involved. Consider drawing the fracture and writing date of immobilization on the cast or splint or, if available, giving patients a copy of their x-rays.

Orthopedic Injuries Common in Children

- *Physeal fracture or Salter-Harris fracture*—fractures involving the physis or growth plate account for 18-30% of pediatric fractures. The cartilaginous composition of the physis makes it weaker and more vulnerable to injuries than tendons or ligaments. This is particularly true during times of rapid adolescent growth. Most common sites of physeal fractures are distal radius, ulna, tibia, and fibula. Sprains are unusual in children with open physes.

- *Buckle or torus fracture*—fracture that involves only a bending of the cortex, resulting from compressive forces. Distal radius and ulna are the most common sites.

- *Bowing or plastic deformity fracture*—excessively bowed bone without radiographic evidence of cortical disruption.

- *Greenstick fracture*—fracture of only one cortex of the diaphysis or metaphysis at the opposite side of the force of impact.

- *Clavicle fracture*—one of the most common fractures of childhood. Shoulder injuries in children are rare. Treatment in the vast majority of cases is sling and swathe immobilization.

- *Supracondylar fracture*—**any fracture involving the distal humerus is considered an orthopedic emergency.** Supracondylar fractures have the greatest risk of any fracture of long-term compromise in function and/or neurovascular injury. The patient will usually hold the arm pronated and resist elbow flexion secondary to pain. A careful neurovascular exam is imperative, because there can be damage to the brachial artery. A pulseless radial artery requires immediate fracture reduction. Long-term risk of neurovascular impairment is higher for supracondylar fractures than any other fractures. The patient should be immobilized and evaluated by an orthopedic surgeon as soon as possible.

- *Nursemaid's or pulled elbow*—caused most commonly by traction on the outstretched elbow. It is an injury in which the radial head subluxes with respect to the annular ligament. It most commonly occurs in infants. The arm is held in partial flexion. Diagnosis is clinical based on history and exam consistent for the condition. In nearly all cases, supination followed by flexion in one rapid motion or hyperpronation with or without flexion corrects the deformity, and most children begin using the arm within 15 minutes.

- *Femur fracture*—blood loss with femur fracture can be clinically significant in children. Traction splinting may be indicated.

- *Toddler's fracture*—spiral fracture of the tibia caused by torque of the lower leg.

FIELD OBSERVATION

Supracondylar fractures are the most common elbow fracture in pediatric patients and usually result from a fall onto an outstretched arm.

Critical Illnesses

Infectious Diseases

The unsanitary environment and crowded conditions in a disaster area increase the risk of serious bacterial illnesses, particularly in children less than 2 years of age and those who have not been immunized. Pediatric patients are often the first to exhibit manifestations of enteritis. **Oral rehydration should be attempted as initial therapy for mild to moderate dehydration.**

Meningitis may result from head trauma such as basilar skull fractures and/or crowded, unsanitary conditions. Empiric antibiotic treatment and, when clinically indicated, cardiorespiratory support should be given. Family members of patients with meningitis should receive prophylaxis as appropriate based on the likely pathogen.

Medication Emergencies

The disrupted disaster environment with limited supervision often results in ingestion of medications, particularly in crowded shelter situations. Additionally, children dependent upon medications to control their disease states may no longer have access to them, resulting in emergencies such as status asthmaticus and status epilepticus.

Heat and Cold Emergencies

A disrupted environment without adequate protection from the elements puts children at a significant risk for both heat illnesses and hypothermia. Establishing and maintaining normal body temperature is essential for body homeostasis, to maintain cardiac and neurologic function, and to prevent coagulopathy. **In comparison to adults, young children have a higher body surface area to mass ratio.** Thinner skin, less subcutaneous tissue, and greater body surface area to mass ratio result in a greater impact of heat and cold on children. Children are also more susceptible to heat illnesses as they become dehydrated more quickly than adults.

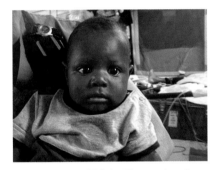

Fig. 15.11 Child with moderate dehydration treated with oral rehydration therapy, Haiti earthquake (2010)

Care of pediatric disaster victims should include cooling and warming as their condition requires. Maintaining and restoring normal body temperature can be challenging given limited resources, particularly in austere environments. At a minimum, heat illness should be treated with cool wet cloths and, as available, fans and ice. Cold illness can be treated with IV fluids warmed near generators and space blankets.

Exposure to Biological, Radioactive and Chemical Agents

Children are more likely to be the first to manifest symptoms from aerosolized biological, radioactive, and chemical agents because of increased respiratory rate and minute volume. In addition, many of these agents, particularly radioactive particles and nerve gases, are denser than oxygen, and thus settle closer to the ground at the level where children breathe.

Thinner cutaneous layers and greater body surface area to mass also increase exposure. In the neonate and very young infant, an immature immune system and lack of full immunization increases the risk of serious illness from biologic agents.

Newborn Delivery and Resuscitation

Births are often increased during a disaster because of physical, psychosocial, and environmental stressors that induce early labor. Neonatal Advanced Life Support guidelines, developed by the AHA, should be followed for care of the newborn on delivery. Neonatal resuscitation requires warming, clearing of the airway, drying, stimulating, and administering vitamin K to prevent hemorrhagic disease of the newborn and erythromycin eye ointment to prevent sexually transmitted ocular infection. Further care is dictated by maternal history and condition of the newborn.

Summary

Medical providers face significant challenges in the care of pediatric illnesses and/or traumatic injuries in a disaster situation, especially in austere environments. Dehydration, infectious diseases, orthopedic injuries, and climate-related illnesses are frequent in children affected by disasters. Knowledge of the unique requirements for assessment, resuscitation, and care of specific injuries is key to the successful care of children in disasters.

KEY POINTS

Most cardiac arrests in children are the result of respiratory compromise. Bradypnea is an ominous late sign of respiratory distress in children.

Dosing tapes are a valuable adjunct in the care of pediatric patients, providing equipment sizes and medication doses based on patient length as a proxy for weight. Weight estimates may require adjustments in non-US settings.

Children are particularly susceptible to climate-related heat and cold illnesses.

Children are more sensitive to aerosolized biological, radioactive, and chemical agents.

Obstetrical Care in Disasters

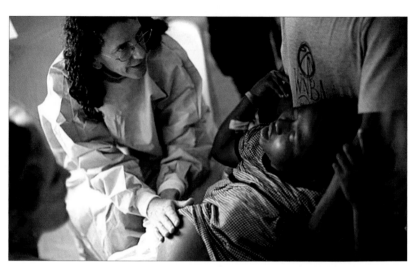

Fig. 16.1 Pregnant patient with preeclampsia (Haiti, 2010).

CASE SCENARIO

Prior to the devastating 7.0 earthquake on January 12, 2010, the impoverished country of Haiti had a significantly high infant mortality rate of 63-68 deaths/1,000 live births according to United Nations estimates (2005-2010). Deficiencies in prenatal, perinatal and postnatal care in many areas of the country contributed to high infant and maternal mortality and morbidity rates. Following the earthquake, care of infants and mothers was a high priority.

Introduction

A disaster setting brings special challenges to the management of a pregnant woman. The normal physiologic changes of pregnancy can place a woman in a particularly vulnerable position. Even a normal pregnancy and labor has risks of pregnancy loss and maternal death in a disaster setting, due to secondary issues of dehydration, nutritional deprivation, and an austere environment.

Normal Pregnancy

A normal full-term pregnancy is 40 weeks (nine months) from the date of the woman's last menstrual period (LMP). It is conventionally divided into three trimesters, each roughly three months long. The three trimesters are distinct periods in which different phases of fetal development take place.

First Trimester (Weeks 1-13)

First trimester is the time of major organogenesis. Women in this trimester may experience nausea from the elevated levels of estrogen and progesterone. **Excessive nausea or vomiting during this time is called *hyperemesis gravidarum*.** Treatment of the condition may require intravenous hydration.

The normal growth of the uterus during the first trimester can be assessed by pelvic examination. On speculum exam, the cervix will be edematous and bluish. The size of the uterus can be measured by bimanual pelvic examination. **The uterus is an intrapelvic organ until approximately the twelth week.** A 12 week pregnancy is a grapefruit size, and the uterus can be palpated at the pubic bone. Around 10-12 weeks of pregnancy, fetal heart tones can be ascertained by doptone. A normal heart rate at this gestation is 120 to 180 beats per minute (bpm) with an average of 150 bpm.

During this trimester, exposure to certain drugs and radiation can induce miscarriages or birth defects. Common teratogenic medications in pregnancy include, but are not limited to:

- Angiotensin-converting-enzyme (ACE) inhibitors
- Carbamazepine
- Cocaine
- Coumadin
- Ethanol
- Isotretinoin
- Lithium
- Methimazole
- Methotrexate
- Misoprostol
- Phenytoin
- Tamoxifen
- Thalidomide
- Valproic acid

179

Second Trimester (Weeks 14-27)

The second trimester is a time of active maturation of the nervous system, the lungs and the gut. **Fetal movement is usually felt by the mother by 17-21 weeks in multiparas and 19-21 weeks in nulliparas.** The position of the uterus at 16 weeks is about halfway between the pubic bone and the umbilicus (with an empty bladder). At 20 weeks, the top of the uterus (fundal height) is at the umbilicus. After 20 weeks, the fundal height increases by 1cm or fingerbreadth above the umbilicus per week.

Third Trimester (Weeks 28-40)

The third trimester is a time of active fetal growth and continued maturation of all organ systems. Depending on medical resources, the ability of a premature baby to survive will vary. In a country with a well-developed medical system, fetal viability is 80% at 26 weeks. **In austere environments or disaster settings without adequate medical resources, there is a high risk of neonatal death for infants born before 34 weeks.**

Major Maternal Complications by Trimester

TOOLS FOR EVALUATION

- Tape measure
- Dating wheel
- Blood pressure (BP) cuff
- Stethoscope
- Fetoscope/doptone
- Portable ultrasound
- Urine dipstick
- ISTAT
- Nitrazine paper
- Sterile gloves

Trimester	Weeks of Pregnancy	Maternal Complications
I	0-13	Bleeding, hyperemesis gravidarum
II	14-27	Bleeding, preeclampsia/eclampsia after 20 weeks
III	28-40	Premature delivery, preeclampsia/eclampsia

Physical Exam of the Pregnant Patient

- Maternal vital signs
- Palpation of the abdomen
- Measure fundal height
- Ascertain if uterine size is appropriate for dates **(Naegele's Rule: Last day of normal menses + 7 days – 3 months + 1 year)**
- Pelvic exam to assess for uterine enlargement
- Check for fetal heart beat

Normal Physiologic Changes in Pregnancy

The following are normal physiologic changes in a pregnant female:

- Heart rate increased by 10-15 beats/minute
- Blood pressure decreased by 5-15 mm Hg in first and second trimesters due to decreased peripheral vascular resistance
- Increase in plasma volume, leading to physiologic anemia of pregnancy
- Increase in cardiac output; 20 to 30% of cardiac output goes to uterus and placenta
- Respiratory alkalosis
- Delayed gastric emptying

Medical Problems of Pregnancy

Preeclampsia

Preeclampsia is a condition in pregnancy characterized by the following:

- Abrupt onset of hypertension
- Proteinuria
- Most common complication of pregnancy
- Usually occurs after 20 weeks' gestation

Risk Factors for Preeclampsia

- Extremes of reproductive age (<20 or >35)
- First pregnancy
- Multiple pregnancies
- Hydatidiform mole
- Family history
- Pre-existing hypertension, renal disease, or diabetes
- Maternal obesity
- Previous severe, early-onset preeclampsia

Severe preeclampsia is characterized by the following:

- BP greater or equal to 160 mm Hg systolic or diastolic greater or equal to 110 on 2 occasions 6 hours apart while patient is at bed rest; and/or headache, right upper quadrant pain, epigastric pain
- Proteinuria greater or equal to 5 grams/24-hour collection or 3+ on dipstick of 2 samples 4 hours apart
- Oliguria less than 500mL/24 hours
- Pulmonary edema or cyanosis
- Impaired liver function
- Thrombocytopenia
- Fetal growth restriction

RISK ALERT!

A pregnant woman in the supine position may exhibit hypotension due to compression of the inferior vena cava.

Position pregnant patient in left lateral position or sitting, if possible.

RISK ALERT!

Pregnant patients with preeclampsia can develop HELLP Syndrome: hemolysis, elevated liver enzymes, low platelets, and severe coagulopathies.

Management of Preeclampsia

- Close monitoring of vital signs (BP)
- Anti-hypertensive medication
- Magnesium sulfate
- Delivery (induction of labor or C-section)

Eclampsia

- Eclampsia involves convulsions (tonic-clonic seizures) in pregnancy not attributable to any other causes such as epilepsy, meningitis, central nervous system (CNS) tumors, head injury, or electrolyte abnormalities.
- **Usually, but not always, preceded by signs and symptoms of preeclampsia.**

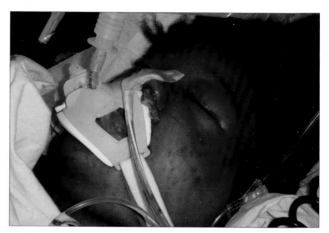

Fig. 16.2 Pregnant patient presenting with eclampsia and seizures, Haiti earthquake (2010)

Management of Eclampsia

- Control seizures
- Control blood pressure
- Immediate delivery

Gestational Diabetes

Gestational diabetes mellitus (GDM) is characterized by carbohydrate intolerance of variable severity with onset of first presentation in pregnancy.

Risk Factors for GDM

- Previous GDM
- Family history of diabetes
- Previous macrosomic (big) baby
- Previous unexplained stillbirth
- Obesity
- Glycosuria
- Polyhydramnios (excess of amniotic fluid in amniotic sac)
- Large for gestation age (LGA) in the current pregnancy

Management of GDM

- Dietary modification, including calorie reduction
- Insulin if persistent fasting or postprandial hyperglycemia
- Intrapartum fetal monitoring
- Ultrasound scan to monitor fetal growth

Bleeding

- Miscarriage: incomplete/complete/septic abortion
- Labor and delivery: vaginal and perianal lacerations, uterine inversion after delivery, uterine rupture
- Placental pathology
- Trauma
- Cancer: cervix, vagina, gestational trophoblastic
- Coagulopathy: sepsis, medications

Tumors

- Benign
- Malignant

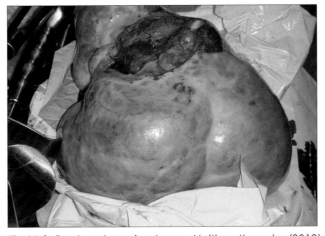

Fig.16.3 Ruptured ovarian tumor, Haiti earthquake (2010)

Infection

- Pregnant women are more vulnerable to infections, and the consequences can be more severe than in the non-pregnant female.

- Viral illnesses and simple upper respiratory tract infections can be more severe, leading to dehydration and secondary pneumonia.

- Urinary tract infections are more common as pregnancy progresses, and as the ureters are compressed by the enlarging uterus, leading to pyelonephritis.

- Dehydration and infection can lead to premature labor.

Seizures

- Assume eclampsia in the absence of head trauma.

- Place patient on left side.

- Protect airway.

- Administer magnesium (6 gm bolus, 2 gm/hour following initial dose).

- Following stabilization, proceed with C-section or induction with oxytocin.

Ectopic Pregnancy

An ectopic pregnancy is a pregnancy that is not in the uterus. The fertilized egg settles and grows in any location other than the inner lining of the uterus. The large majority (95%) of ectopic pregnancies occur in the Fallopian tubes. However, they can occur in other locations, such as the ovary, cervix, and abdominal cavity.

Placental Problems in Utero

Problem	Cause	Diagnosis	Intervention
Placentia Previa (implantation of placenta over cervical opening)	Prior C-section, dilatation and curettage (D&C), multiple pregnancies	Copious, painless vaginal bleeding; Ultrasound	C-section if complete previa. Vaginal delivery is possible with marginal previa if the mother and fetus are stable.
Abruptio Placentae (premature separation of placenta from uterus). This condition is associated with hemorrhage between the placenta and the uterine wall which leads to contractions and premature delivery.	Direct blunt trauma to uterus, cardiovascular disease, smoking, multiple gestations, cocaine use	Bleeding, pain, rigid abdomen	C-section Vaginal delivery may be possible if mother and fetus are stable, and delivery is very close or imminent.

Labor and Delivery

Delivery Area

The delivery area, in either mobile or fixed medical facilities, should be located in a quiet area out of general traffic. Use barricades such as sheets to cordon off an area and shield the patient, if possible. Changing the patient out of her street clothes is important, not just for cleanliness, but for another important consideration. Following a disaster, the clothing the patient is wearing may be the only ones she has left.

In an emergency, delivery can be accomplished on the ground, but it is much easier if the patient can be delivered on a raised platform. A bed is optimal, but a stretcher supported on a stable base or a table are reasonable alternatives.

Labor

Determination of actual labor versus false labor in the presenting obstetrical patient is the same in disasters as in non-disaster settings, but the techniques of evaluation may require modification. A cervical exam to determine change in dilatation and palpation of the abdomen to determine strength of contractions are essential.

There are three stages of labor. During the first stage (called the stage of dilatation), the cervix dilates fully to a diameter of about 10 cm. In the second stage (called the stage of expulsion), the baby moves out through the cervix and vagina to be born. The third stage is the time period after delivery of the neonate until the delivery of the placenta has been accomplished.

There are several ways to assess the patient if there is a suspicion of leaking amniotic fluid.

- One may observe fluid coming from the vaginal introitus alone or coming out of the cervix during a speculum exam. **(The Valsalva maneuver may be useful if no fluid is seen initially pooling in the vagina or coming from the cervical os.)**
- Nitrazine paper can help in rendering a presumptive diagnosis of ruptured membranes. This test reflects the pH of the fluid. The vagina normally has a pH of 4.5-7.5. Amniotic fluid has a pH of 7.0-7.5.

Delivery of the Newborn Child

Most births are uncomplicated, and spontaneous delivery can usually be accomplished. Ease of delivery will depend on several factors: number of prior deliveries, gestational age of infant, and position of the fetus in the uterus.

Position of Fetus in Utero

Position	Description	Delivery complications
Vertex	Head down	Vaginal delivery
Breech	Buttocks down	Vaginal delivery possible if frank or complete breech; C-Section if incomplete breech
Transverse lie	Back down	C-Section

Vertex presentation:
The vertex or fetal head is facing the birth canal.

Breech presentation:
The 3 types of breech presentation are as follows:

- Frank (65%): Hips of the fetus are flexed, and knees are extended.
- Complete (10%): The hips and knees of the fetus are flexed.
- Incomplete (25%): The feet or knees of the fetus are the lowermost presenting part.

    o Single footling: One of the lower extremities is lowermost.

    o Double footling: Both of the lower extremities are lowermost.

Transverse presentation:
- The fetal back is facing the birth canal.

Vaginal Delivery

General Procedure

The general procedure for vaginal delivery is as follows:

- Swab the perineum with povidone iodophor and drape it with towels. **Control the baby's head with the nondominant hand.** If necessary to permit delivery of the baby, inject the midline perineum with lidocaine, and perform a midline incision down to (but not into) the rectal muscle. Usually, the amniotic sac has broken; if not, open it now. Note the color and consistency of the amniotic fluid.

- **Once the head emerges, suction the mouth and nose.** Use a bulb syringe if excessive sections are present.

- **Check the neonate's neck for the umbilical cord.** If it is wrapped around the neck, pull it gently over the head. If this is not possible (e.g., it is too tight or has too many loops), double clamp the cord and divide the cord between the clamps. Recheck the neck because the cord may be wrapped around the neck more than once. Deliver the child expeditiously.

- **Gentle traction toward the mother's posterior usually delivers the anterior shoulder.** If this attempt is unsuccessful, try pressing down over the mother's bladder to move the anterior shoulder posteriorly. If this is unsuccessful, shoulder dystocia may be present. A number of options to address this exist, including delivering the posterior shoulder, rotating the anterior shoulder posteriorly, and then delivering that shoulder.

- Once the shoulders are out, the rest of the baby slips out quickly. Be careful because neonates are slippery. Keep the nondominant hand in place, controlling the baby's head, and slide the dominant hand under and along the baby as it emerges. Once the feet are out, rotate the baby 180° into a football hold. Suction the nose and mouth. **Double clamp the cord 7-10 cm from the baby, and cut the cord between the clamps.**

- If the child starts breathing and moving and appears to be in good health, turn the baby over to nursing personnel. Make sure that the baby is vigorously dried, suctioned, and kept warm. **If the birth is complicated by thick meconium (amniotic fluid that is thick and pea green), do not stimulate the baby to cry.** Instead, use a 3.0 endotracheal tube to intubate the trachea, suction the child, and stimulate the baby's breathing.

ESSENTIAL SUPPLIES FOR VAGINAL DELIVERY

- Suction tubing
- Needle driver
- Scissors
- Sutures
- Kelly clamps
- Sterile gauze
- Gloves
- Bulb syringe
- Warming blanket
- Dry towels

- Clamping of the umbilical cord can be accomplished with surgical clamps or suture, if available. The umbilical cord can also be tied off with a string (sterile, if available). Feel the top of the uterus. If it is almost in the pelvis, it is probable that only one fetus exists. **Be sure another fetus is not present prior to delivery of the placenta.**

- Allow the third stage of labor, delivery of the placenta, to proceed slowly. **Delivery of the placenta will usually take place spontaneously. Do not pull on the cord.** Guide the placenta out as it is expelled, and inspect the placenta to ensure that it is entirely expelled. **Excessive pulling on the cord can lead to snapping it off or uterine inversion, which can result in extreme blood loss.**

- As soon as the cord has been cut, if no resuscitation is required, place the neonate directly onto the mother's chest, skin to skin, to enable the neonate to maintain his/her body temperature. Do not neglect drying off the neonate while on the mother's chest. If left wet, neonates can lose a large amount of heat, causing complications.

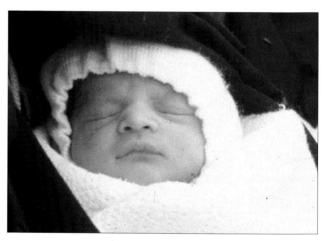

Fig.16.4 Delivery of healthy newborn,
Iran earthquake (2004)

- Other methods of keeping neonates warm after delivery include use of a small plastic bag. Cut a hole in the bottom of the bag for the head and place the bag on the neonate like a gown without arm holes to trap body heat, thereby allowing maintenance of appropriate temperature. Placing a neonate in a small cardboard box as a bassinet is also helpful. The use of space blankets or even plastic wrap over the box, with a space for air, can also be beneficial. Warm intravenous (IV) bags in the box next to the neonate can also help. Care must be taken to constantly monitor the neonate when using all alternative warming devices.

- **In a disaster, keeping wounds to a minimum is important and routine episiotomy is not recommended.** Routine use of episiotomy often results in more complications than lacerations alone.

- Apgar scoring is used to provide a rough estimate of the baby's immediate adaptation to extrauterine life. The score aids in determination of whether the baby is viable independently or needs help (resuscitation). Apgar scores should be documented at 1, 5, and 10 minutes in all neonates. If the 5-minute score is less than 7, continue scoring every 5 minutes for 20 minutes. However, if the child requires resuscitation, waiting to do a 1-minute score is not indicated.

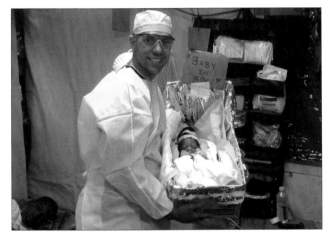

*Fig.16.5 Newborn baby in cardboard box,
Haiti earthquake (2010)*

Assign scores in each of the following categories and total them for the Apgar score.

APGAR Score

Sign	Score = 0	Score = 1	Score = 2
Appearance	Blue or pale	Body pink, limbs blue	Pink all over
Heart Rate	Absent	<100 bpm	>100 bpm
Grimace	No response	Some motion	Crying
Activity	Limp	Some weak motion	Active
Respiration	None	Weak cry	Strong cry

Neonatal Resuscitation in the Field

- Erythromycin ointment or gentamycin 2 drops to both eyes

- Vitamin K 1 mg intramuscular (IM)

- Ampicillin 50 mg/kg IM if maternal temperature greater than 38° C, rupture of membranes greater than 18 hours, or gestation less than 37 weeks

- Test mother for HIV. If positive, AZT (zidovudine) 4 mg/kg bid for 6 weeks

- In disaster environments, consider tetanus immune globulin if mother has never been immunized or has had no booster in 10 years.

Postpartum Care

The possibility of postpartum hemorrhage is most profound during the period immediately following the birth. The amount of vaginal bleeding should be carefully monitored. If it increases, massaging the uterus will usually cause the myometrium to contract and slow bleeding. It may also help expel clots that may be forming in the endometrial cavity. If a vaginal hematoma is observed and is stable, conservative treatment is recommended.

The vulva and perineum can be quite tender for a few days following delivery, and the use of ice packs for the first 24 hours may help alleviate discomfort, if available. Care must be taken to monitor the patient's ability to void after delivery.

> ## SPECIAL RISKS DURING THE POSTPARTUM PERIOD
> - Hemorrhage
> - Vaginal hematomas
> - Urinary retention
> - Infection
> - Pulmonary embolus

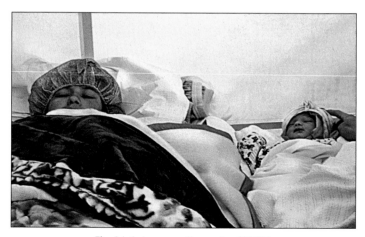

Fig.16.6 Iran earthquake (2003)

190

Complications of Delivery

Obstructed Labor

Obstructed labor can occur because of fetal macrosomia, twins or higher multiples, or abnormal presentation of fetus.

Premature Labor

The most common reason for preterm labor is dehydration. Other causes include infection, multiple gestations, trauma, smoking, and some drugs.

Umbilical Cord Accidents

Problem	Cause	Diagnosis	Intervention
Cord compression with contractions	Reduced amniotic volume	Decreased fetal heart rate	Delivery
Cord prolapse	Ruptured membranes	Cord in vagina in front of fetal head	Manually push back fetal head and urgent C-section
Transverse or breech position			Urgent C-section
Cord around fetal neck	Common occurrence	Manual palpation during delivery	Remove or cut cord
True knot	Unknown	Decreased fetal heart rate with contractions	Delivery; possible urgent C-section

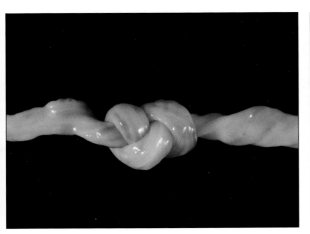 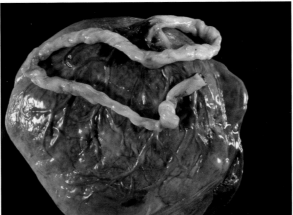

Figs. 16.7, 16.8 True knots in umbilical cords

191

Cesarean Section

- Prep abdomen.
- Place Foley catheter.
- Incise midline from umbilicus to symphysis pubis (or perform a Pfannenstiel incision, which can reduce postoperative pain and dehiscence incidence).
- Separate rectus muscle; avoid bowel/bladder.
- Incise uterus transversely in the lower uterine segment with care to avoid lateral vessels.
- Deliver infant and placenta.
- Close uterus with layered closure (delayed absorbable suture).
- Close fascia and skin.
- Administer antibiotics concurrently: third generation cephalosporin, clindamycin, ampicillin, and gentamicin are all effective.

In the unfortunate circumstance it is necessary to perform a perimortum Cesarean section to save the life of the fetus, the procedure should be performed after 4 minutes of attempted resuscitation of the mother or if maternal death is imminent and fetus is greater than 24 weeks.

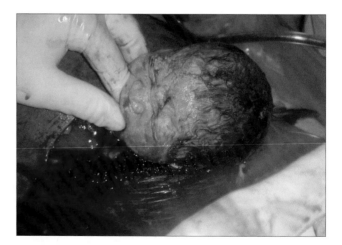

Fig.16.8 Cesarean section, Haiti earthquake (2010)

Intubation in Pregnant Patients

Pregnant women have a laxity of the gastroesophageal sphincter and prolonged intestinal transit time, which leads to an increased risk of aspiration. Treatment should include:

- Administer an antacid, if available, prior to intubation.
- Rapid sequence induction is recommended with succinylcholine, ketamine, propofol, or etomidate.
- Low-dose inhaled anesthetics may be used but can cause uterine atony.
- Fentanyl and narcotics are recommended post-delivery of the uterus.

Summary

In the wake of a disaster, medical personnel are faced with a unique set of circumstances in the care of pregnant patients. In addition to the stresses of the pregnancy and subsequent delivery of the newborn child, the woman may have lost her home, belongings, and even some of her family members. Privacy and respect for pregnant women are of prime importance. Cultural awareness should not be forgotten, even in the chaos of the disaster.

KEY POINTS

 Preeclampsia is the most common complication of pregnancy and usually, but not always, precedes the onset of eclampsia.

 Pregnant women in the SUPINE position may have significant compression of the inferior vena cava in the last trimester. If hypotensive, immediately position the patient in the left lateral position to relieve compression.

 Pregnant women have a physiologic increase in cardiac output, which may mask early signs of hypovolemic shock.

 In the absence of head trauma, assume eclampsia in a pregnant patient in the last trimester presenting with seizures.

Extremity Injuries

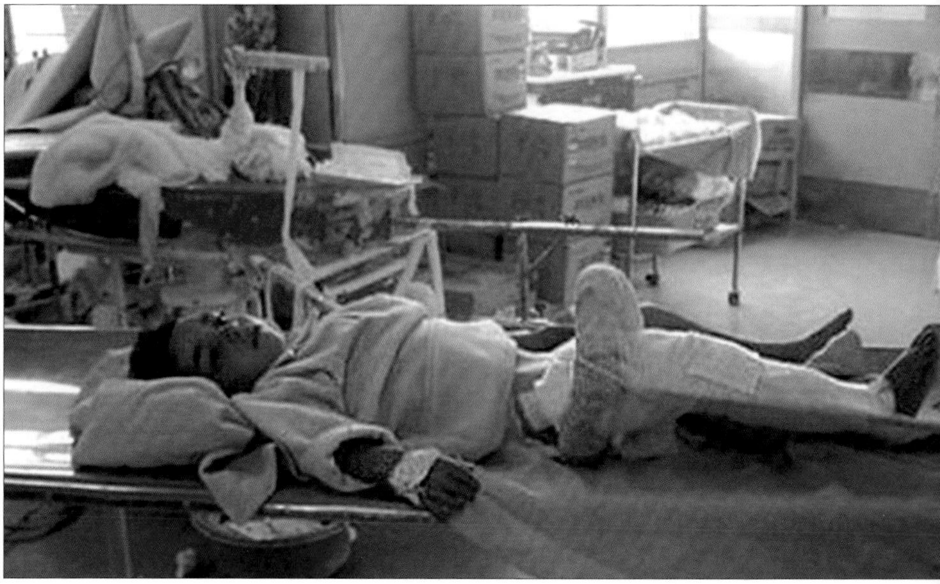

Fig.17.1 Pakistan earthquake (2005)

CASE SCENARIO

On October 8, 2005, a devastating earthquake occurred in the Pakistan-administered region of Kashmir. The 7.6 earthquake, similar in size to the 1906 San Francisco earthquake, killed over 75,000 individuals and injured over 106,000 victims. The remote geographic region complicated the logistics of providing disaster relief and evacuating casualties to hospitals throughout Pakistan. Teams from throughout the world provided disaster medical relief and supplies. Orthopedic injuries were common in surviving casualties.

Introduction

Most disasters, whether natural or man-made events, cause significant numbers of musculoskeletal injuries. Most orthopedic injuries are not life- threatening and should not divert attention from treatment of other potentially lethal injuries. Some injuries, however, require prompt treatment for control of hemorrhage.

Triage

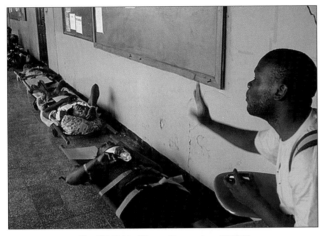

Fig.17.2 Haiti earthquake (2010)

Triage must often be done quickly in disasters due to the large number of victims presenting for medical care. Four primary categories of orthopedic injuries can be identified:

- Patients who require immediate treatment
- Patients in whom a delay is acceptable
- The minimally injured ("walking wounded")
- Non-salvageable patients due to severity of injuries or lack of resources ("expectant" category of victims)

The concept of **"damage control orthopedics"** (temporizing severe musculoskeletal injuries in potentially salvageable casualties) is applicable in the first and second groups. The latter two require little or no formal orthopedic care at the disaster scene.

Initial Assessment

- Cut away clothing as necessary to allow for proper observation of skin contusions, abrasions, lacerations, or bleeding.

- Systematically evaluate the upper and lower extremities. If the victim is awake, he/she may be able to assist by indicating primary areas of pain.

- Note non-anatomical or inappropriate positioning of the extremity.

- Note any tenderness, crepitation, joint instability, or abnormal motion of the extremity.

PRIMARY MANAGEMENT OF EXTREMITY TRAUMA

- **Control of hemorrhage**
- **Neurological/vascular assessment**
- **Realign gross deformities/obvious dislocations**
- **Irrigate and dress open wounds**
- **Splinting**

Control of Hemorrhage

Control of hemorrhage is the first priority and can often be slowed by direct pressure or the use of hemostatic agents such as combat gauze. Do not attempt blind clamping of bleeding vessels. **Tourniquets have proven life-saving and should be used for control of exsanguinating extremity hemorrhage. If a tourniquet is required, attach a tag to the device, noting the time of application.** Blast injuries with traumatic amputations often require tourniquet application.

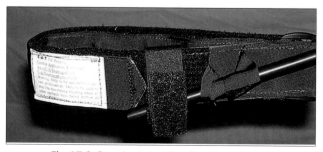

Fig. 17.3 Combat Application Tourniquet, Courtesy of Department of Defense

Pelvic fractures are a less obvious cause of hemorrhage, but can be just as lethal. They should be diagnosed by pain and tenderness in responsive victims and instability of the pelvis in obtunded victims. Patients suspected of having a pelvic fracture need to be splinted with a back board and wrapped in a pelvic binder (pelvic wrap) to improve pelvic stability and decrease ongoing blood loss. **Pelvic binder should be wrapped at the level of the hips.**

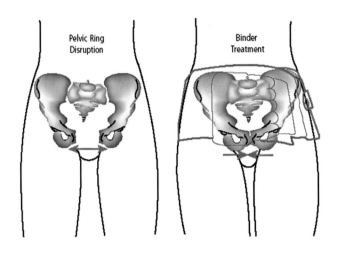

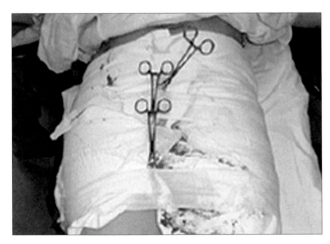

Fig.17.4 Pelvic Binder

Vascular/Neurological Examination

Following control of hemorrhage, all injured limbs should be assessed for pulses, neurological deficits, and painful swelling. These indicate a time-sensitive diagnosis (vascular injury, nerve impingement, or compartment syndrome). If vascular or neurological deficits exist, combined with a skeletal or joint deformity in the limb, a reduction of the deformity should be done judiciously with traction along the overall axis of the limb. A simple splint should be applied quickly if immediate transport is necessary or the limb splinted by laying it next to the victim's torso. **If pulses in the injured limb remain absent or decreased asymmetrically, a vascular injury should be suspected and fasciotomy performed at the time of vascular repair or shunting. If possible, vascular repair should be done in less than 6 hours from the onset of the injury.** If this cannot be done, the risk of eventual amputation increases significantly.

Any injury to the extremities has the potential to cause a compartment syndrome (increased pressure within an osteofascial muscle compartment). Skeletal muscle in the extremities is typically invested in fascial compartments that are non-extensible. Following traumatic injury (e.g., crush injury) or after a period of loss of perfusion (e.g., vascular injury), muscle within compartments can swell, causing compartment syndrome. **Compartment syndrome is a surgical emergency. The key to successful treatment of compartment syndrome is early diagnosis and fasciotomy.** Fasciotomies done after the fact or days later may not be prudent as muscle is probably already dead, and this may expose the patient to infection.

Fasciotomy is the prophylactic release of skin and muscle fasciae to relieve pressure in the muscle compartments. If untreated promptly, compartment syndrome can cause secondary muscle injury and necrosis, vascular compromise, and neural injury. Instruments are available to directly measure intracompartmental pressures, but their use may not be practical in a disaster setting. Ultimately, the decision to undertake early compartment decompression should be made based on clinical signs and symptoms. Compartment releases should be done if the limb swelling is accompanied by paresthesias, pain with passive stretching of the affected muscle, or diminished or loss of pulses after attempts at reduction and alignment. **It is generally recommended that erring on the side of performing a fasciotomy is preferable to missing the diagnosis of compartment syndrome.**

In the upper extremity, the forearm and hand are at the highest risk for compartment syndrome. The upper arm may also be at risk for increased compartment pressures. In the lower extremity, the anterior and lateral compartments of the lower leg are at highest risk for increased compartment pressures. The gluteus and thigh may also develop compartment syndrome.

Wound Debridement

Open extremity wounds should be copiously irrigated as soon as possible to remove visible contamination. Drinkable water is equally effective as sterile saline as an irrigating solution. Discard avascular bone fragments as the non-viable surfaces will support bacterial colonization.

- All wounds should be left open due to potential contamination.

- Administer antibiotics, intravenously if possible, against both gram-positive and gram-negative bacteria.

- Administer tetanus booster if date of last booster is unknown. In many low-income countries, vaccination to prevent tetanus is uncommon so tetanus prophylaxis must include immunoglobulin.

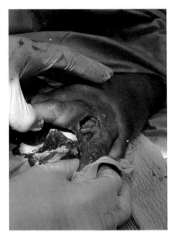 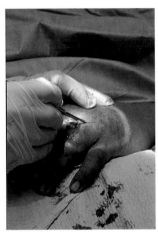

Figs. 17.5, 17.6 Crush Injury of hand with secondary infection, Iran earthquake (2005)

Splinting

The mechanical requirement for splinting is dictated by the need for mobility. If transport is available and the victim can be moved on a litter, the splint can be the victim's body with the lower limbs tied together or the upper limbs swathed to the chest. If the victim must move himself, the splint must be constructed with far more strength and durability.

Spinal injuries necessitate special mobility needs. It should be assumed that obtunded victims must be moved using multiple rescuers and large space-occupying equipment (back boards). Other injuries that should alert rescuers to the possibility of an associated spine injury are calcaneus, periarticular knee, hip, and pelvis fractures after a fall mechanism. In such patients, taking the more difficult steps of moving the victims as if they have an unstable spine (back board) should be considered, even in those who are alert and deny tenderness.

Important principles of splinting include the following:

- Splints should be non-circumferential to allow for swelling
- Splints should extend a joint above and below the injury
- Traction splints for femur fractures provide stabilization, improve comfort, and may prevent further vascular injury. **Note the time of application of the traction splint.**

External Fixation

External fixation in a mass casualty setting is a valuable therapeutic modality in some cases. It is far more likely, however, that initial stabilization of injured extremities or an unstable pelvis will be accomplished by means of splints or external binders. They can be more easily and rapidly applied than even the simplest external skeletal frames, and they are usually quite sufficient to safely evacuate patients to a nearby treatment facility. However, there are instances where external fixation may be preferable, and it is relatively easy to apply for both open and closed fractures.

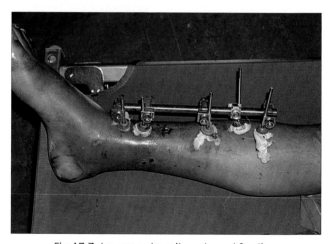

Fig.17.7 Lower extremity external fixation

External fixation has become the mainstay of operative temporization for severe long bone and joint injury, particularly when there is associated soft tissue injury. Other conditions in which external fixation may be useful include:

- Unstable pelvic ring injuries not adequately controlled with an external binder
- Femur fractures with prolonged transport time
- Open extremity fractures with circumferential wounds needing dressing changes
- Extremity fractures with associated vascular injuries
- Extremity fractures at risk for compartment syndrome
- Grossly unstable knee/ankle dislocations
- Extremity fractures in patients who are in shock, have severe head injury, or major thoracoabdominal injury requiring emergent therapy.
- External fixation can serve as "portable traction" to facilitate patient transport during evacuation.
- External fixators can be used to bridge single bone fractures or can be applied across a joint ("joint-spanning frame") in the event of metaphyseal, intra-articular, or associated joint injury.
- External fixation is commonly used on the tibia, femur, knee, and ankle.

Application of an external fixator is relatively quick, and many systems currently in use are modular to allow for a variety of frame configurations. Pin placement can be done percutaneously and does not require the use of x-ray/fluoroscopy if unavailable.

> **TREATMENT TIP**
>
> Lightweight and sterile/pre-packaged extremity fixator sets are commercially available.

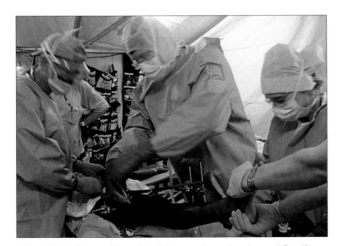

Fig. 17.8 Operative debridement and external fixation of extremity fracture, Haiti earthquake (2010)

Amputation

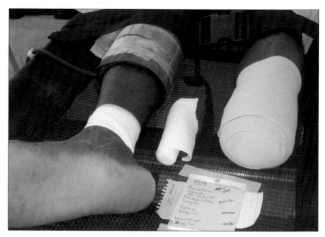

Fig.17.9 Haiti earthquake (2010)

Amputations are frequently required in victims of disasters, especially following blast and crush injuries. Following fractures or dislocations that are accompanied by a pulseless, ischemic limb despite reduction of the malalignment, the incidence of amputation is significantly increased unless a timely vascular repair is possible. Consideration for amputation should be given in the following circumstances:

- To free an entrapped victim (field amputation)
- Severely crushed or mangled extremities
- Prolonged period of ischemia following entrapment
- Refractory bleeding

If amputation is necessary to free an entrapped victim, the amputation should be as distal as possible, with a tourniquet placed above the amputation site. Providers should use the most appropriate and easily available equipment to rapidly amputate the extremity (e.g., handsaw, power saw, surgical instruments, etc). If available, an amputation set that is equipped for both soft tissue and bone resection facilitates field amputations. Preserve as much viable muscle tissue and bone length as possible at the time of primary amputation.

- Take measures to ensure the safety of rescuers.
- Do not "blindly" clamp bleeding vessels, as this may cause injury to adjacent neurovascular structures.
- Ligate major vessels and cut nerves to allow them to retract.
- Dressing the stump open (without wound closure) after vascular ligature is the safest procedure for the patient who is to be evacuated.
- Transverse "guillotine" amputations should be avoided as they are difficult to reconstruct.

Amputation vs. Limb Salvage

Limb salvage vs. amputation is often a difficult decision faced by medical rescuers of disaster victims with mangled limbs. The following clinical findings increase the likelihood that an amputation will ultimately be required:

- High-energy wounds, especially those with gross contamination
- Pulselessness, paresthesia, diminished capillary refill in affected limb(s)
- Cool, paralyzed, insensate, or numb limb(s)
- Persistent hypotension
- Prolonged entrapment with crush injury to soft tissue

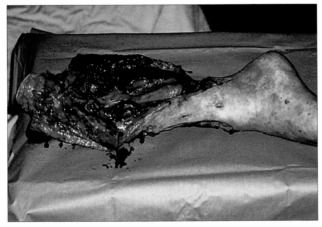

Fig.17.10 Crush injury to leg requiring field amputation

CONTENTS OF FIELD AMPUTATION KIT

- #3 knife handle (1)
- Metzenbaum scissors (1)
- 5" tooth forceps (2)
- Rasp (1)
- Bone cutter (1)
- Straight snap (2)
- Kelly clamp (2)
- Schnidt clamp (2)
- Rongeur
- Wing-tip elevator
- Rake retractor, dull
- Saw
- Tourniquet
- Heavy silk suture

Summary

All limb salvage treatments in disasters must balance risks and benefits. Medical providers responding to disasters globally must have a good sense of what treatments can be sustained locally, as well as the infectious risks of operating in contaminated environments utilizing less than reliable methods to sterilize instruments. This should significantly limit the options a surgeon considers for treatment of orthopedic injuries.

KEY POINTS

 Tourniquets should be used for control of exsanguinating extremity hemorrhage.

 Pelvic binders are an important initial treatment of pelvic fractures to decrease ongoing blood loss.

 Field amputation may be necessary for victim extrication in disasters.

 Compartment syndrome is a surgical emergency requiring immediate fasciotomy.

Eye Injuries

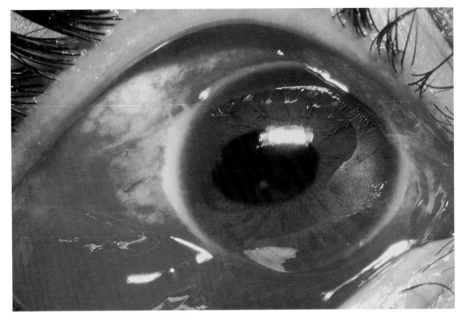

Fig.18.1 *Ruptured globe following severe blunt trauma.*

CASE SCENARIO

Cafés and other public gathering places are favorite targets of terrorists. A terrorist bombing in an outdoor café instantly killed twelve people. Many other victims had secondary blast injuries, including ocular injuries. Eye injuries included <u>blunt trauma</u> (causing disruption of intraocular contents and bleeding, rupture of the globe, abrasions of the surface, and fractures of the periorbital region); <u>lacerating trauma</u> (lacerations of the globe and areas around the eye); and <u>thermal injury</u> (burns of the ocular and periorbital tissues). While awaiting definitive ophthalmic care, basic care includes protecting injured eyes with a patch or shield, cleaning globes and wounds with Normal Saline, administration of Intravenous (IV) antibiotics for ruptured globes, and administration of tetanus prophylaxis as needed.

205

Introduction

Eye injuries are exceedingly common. In a general emergency department, eye injuries and complaints approximate 10% of patient visits. However, the potential for serious vision-threatening injuries greatly exceeds this figure in a natural or man-made disaster.

In any disaster setting, life-threatening injuries take priority and must be managed first. However, it is important to appreciate that eye-related injuries and their sequelae are often long-term problems for disaster survivors. Partial or total blindness in one or both eyes is not uncommon, and cosmetic disfigurement in the periorbital area may be a significant confounding factor. These are lifelong problems with profound physical, psychological, and social effects.

Everyone involved in triage following disasters needs to be able to identify potentially vision-threatening injuries and perform an adequate eye examination. Patients with severe eye injuries need to get immediate emergency treatment to avoid aggravating serious situations until definitive ophthalmic care can be carried out. The focus of this chapter will be on disaster scene triage and stabilization of eye injuries before ophthalmic consultation.

Causes and Mechanisms of Eye Injuries

Blunt Trauma—Blunt assault to the face can occur from fists, weapons, and missiles or objects from any source. Blunt trauma can cause severe disruption of intraocular contents and bleeding, rupture of the globe, abrasions of the surface, and fractures of the periorbital region.

Lacerating Trauma—Knives or any projectile that can be hurled through the air can result in lacerations of the globe or areas around the eye.

Thermal Injury—Explosions with intense heat and/or flame can cause burns of the ocular and periorbital tissues.

Chemical Injury—Foreign chemicals of any type can cause severe damage to the surface of the eye. Alkaline agents, either particulate or liquid in nature, including plaster and lime, are the most damaging.

Photochemical—Focused light, usually in the form of lasers, can cause photochemical and/or photo-thermal injury to the cornea, iris, lens, or retina.

Biological—Depending on the offending agent, symptoms and signs may range from ocular irritation, redness, and swelling to keratitis, uveitis, optic neuritis, retinal vasculitis, and nerve palsies.

Evaluation and Triage of Eye Injuries

History

Obtain a chief complaint directed to the visual system, and amplify by exploring the following areas:

Altered Vision
• Does the patient have blurred vision, double vision, or distorted vision?

Eye Pain
• Does the patient have a foreign-body sensation, sharp pain, or throbbing pain?

Change in Appearance of the Lid/Globe
• Does the patient note swelling, redness, or ocular/orbital discharge?

Trauma
• Characterize the type of injury sustained: Is it blunt, lacerating, explosive, chemical, or foreign-body-related, or a combination of several types?

Previous Eye Problems
• Does the patient have a history of reduced vision or intraocular surgery?

Mechanism of Injury

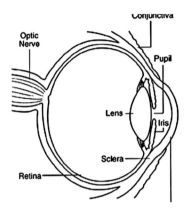

Fig. 18.2
Anatomy of the eye

Eye Examination

Visual Acuity – This is the "vital sign" of the eye.
• Assess visual acuity. A pocket vision card with Snellen equivalents is useful. If vision is significantly reduced to a level below the ability to read print, determine if the patient can count fingers (CF), detect hand motion (HM), or perceive light (PL).

External Examination (Penlight)
• Lids/Orbit—Assess for structural integrity and function. Document presence or absence of swelling, proptosis, ptosis, or discharge. Palpate for orbital fractures.

• Sclera/Conjunctiva—Assess for lacerations, hemorrhage, or foreign bodies. The lid eversion technique is helpful (see opposite).

• Cornea—Assess for structural integrity and foreign bodies. Diagnosis is facilitated by use of topical fluorescein and illumination of the ocular surface with cobalt blue-filtered light.

EXAMINATION TIP:

Lid Eversion Technique

The lid eversion technique is useful for examining the whites of the eyes in the absence of lacerating trauma.

Grasp upper lid eyelashes with one hand and flip the lid up and over a cotton-tipped applicator applied to the lid approximately 10 mm above the lid margin.

Neuro-Medical Examination

- Pupil—Assess for any asymmetry in pupil reactivity, shape, or size. The presence of an afferent pupillary defect is an important sign of optic nerve damage.

- Extraocular Movements—Determine the disaster victim's ability to move both eyes right, left, up, and down.

Ophthalmoscopy

- Use an ophthalmoscope if it is available at the scene to view the optic nerve, retina, and blood vessels. Simple observation of the normal red reflex that is present with the direct ophthalmoscope may also detect the presence of vitreous hemorrhage or retinal detachment.

Intraocular Pressure

- *Acute glaucoma* (elevated intraocular pressure) is very uncommon in disaster settings; therefore, little attention to high intraocular pressure is required. Intraocular pressure may be very low in the setting of globe laceration.

Basic Eye Equipment for Emergency Triage Use

- Pocket vision card with Snellen equivalents
- Magnifying loupes (optional)
- Hand-held illuminator/flashlight
- Cobalt-blue filter
- Cotton-tip applicators
- Direct ophthalmoscope
- Topical anesthetic (e.g., proparacaine, tetracaine)
- Topical fluorescein strips
- Squeeze bottle for ocular-surface irrigation
- Sterile balanced salt solution
- Topical antibiotic drops (ofloxacin, gentamycin, polymyxin/trimethoprim)
- Topical antibiotic ointment (Bacitracin, gentamicin)
- Artificial-tear supplements
- Protective shield
- Eye patches
- Tape
- Basic suture set including #4-0, #6-0 silk; #4-0, #6-0 absorbable sutures

Emergency Treatment of Eye Injuries

Chemical Burns

Chemical burns represent a true vision-threatening emergency. **Alkaline agents are potentially more damaging than acid agents because they more easily penetrate the structure of the eye.** Both alkaline and acid agents can be present in the form of fluids or particulate matter.

Treatment

- Immediately irrigate with any non-toxic fluid—preferably water or Normal Saline (NS). Severe chemical burns may require irrigation with one or more liters of sterile saline or water. Topical anesthetic drops facilitate effective irrigation.

- Remove all particulate matter utilizing the lid eversion technique.

- Administer a topical antibiotic drop or ointment, and close the eyes with tape or patch. Refer promptly to an eye care facility as soon as possible.

Thermal Burns

Thermal burns can be associated with chemical burns, particularly in the setting of explosions. Fortunately, the blink reflex usually protects the eye, but adnexal injury involving the lids and orbit is very common. Associated findings may include:

Incomplete Lid Closure

Incomplete lid closure can occur with significant burns, leading to skin retraction and ectropion.

Treatment

- Lubricate the ocular surface with ophthalmic ointment.

Ocular Surface Burn/Corneal Abrasion

This condition may be detected with application of topical fluorescein and cobalt-blue evaluation of the cornea.

Treatment

- Apply topical antibiotic drops or ointment.
- Close the lids with tape or patch.

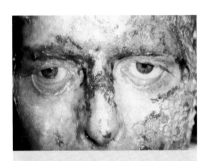

Figure 18.3
Ectropion after facial burn with corneal exposure

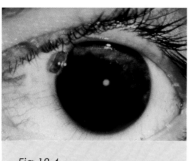

Fig.18.4
Ruptured globe with uveal prolapse and hyphema

TREATMENT ALERT!

Avoid pressure patches in treatment of a ruptured globe. Protect the eye with protective shield only.

Ruptured Globe

This condition generally requires urgent ophthalmic surgical repair. All triage personnel should have a high level of suspicion for ruptured globes, because vision can often be excellent (even 20/20), despite full-thickness globe penetration. Mechanism of injury with high-speed particulate matter (e.g., explosives or metal on metal) should raise the suspicion for a ruptured globe.

Clues to detection include:

* Bullous, elevated subconjunctival hemorrhage
* Conjunctival laceration
* *Uveal prolapse*—extravasation of colored brown iris or choroidal tissue outside the eye
* An irregularly shaped pupil
* *Hyphema*—blood in the anterior chamber
* Lens opacity/traumatic cataract development

Treatment

* Protect the eye with a protective shield—do not patch. If no shield, then a 4 x 4 or a cup can protect the globe.
* Administer tetanus prophylaxis.
* If there will be any delay in definitive surgical care, administer topical antibiotic drops (not ointment) and IV antibiotics, providing gram-positive and gram-negative coverage.
* In the setting of an avulsed eye with severe disruption of ocular and orbital contents, protective-shield placement over the orbital area is indicated.

These patients need prompt transfer to an ophthalmic surgical facility for computed tomography (CT)/possible magnetic resonance imaging (MRI) scanning and definitive surgical repair.

Hyphema

Hyphema, or blood in the anterior chamber, may indicate a ruptured globe and must be treated appropriately if present.

Treatment

In the absence of a ruptured globe, treatment is as follows:

* Protect the eye with a shield.
* Elevate the casualty's head to facilitate gravitational settling of the blood.

Blunt Orbital Trauma

Blunt Trauma without Fracture ("Black Eye")

Findings include:

- *Ecchymosis* (bruising)

- Swelling

- Subconjunctival hemorrhage

Treatment

- Apply cold compresses and refer for routine ophthalmic follow-up.

Retrobulbar Hemorrhage

Findings include:

- Pain

- *Proptosis* (forward protrusion of the eyeball)

- Congestion of orbital tissues

- Reduced vision

Treatment

- Triage immediately to a definitive ophthalmic facility to decompress the eye and orbit.

Orbital Fractures

Orbital fractures are rarely a surgical emergency. Clues to diagnosis of orbital fractures include:

- *Diplopia* (double vision) with restricted extraocular motility

- *Enophthalmos* or *proptosis* (backward or forward displacement)

- Infraorbital nerve *hypoesthesia* (reduced sensitivity)

- Orbital rim step-off or instability

- Orbital *emphysema* (swelling)

- Cerebrospinal fluid *rhinorrhea* (runny nose)

Treatment

- Apply cold compresses.

- Provide appropriate pain relief.

- Administer systemic antibiotics to decrease risk for orbital infection.

- Refer for eye and ear, nose, throat (ENT) evaluation.

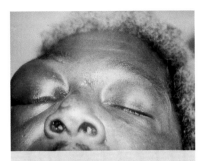

Fig.18.5
Proptosis with lid swelling following blunt trauma.

211

Orbital Foreign Bodies
Treatment
- Assume the globe is ruptured, and treat accordingly.
- Stabilize the foreign body.
- Do <u>not</u> remove orbital foreign bodies. This should be done only under controlled circumstances, and all triage treatment should be directed at prevention of undesired foreign-body movement and migration.

Lacerating Orbital Trauma with Lid Laceration
As with other blunt trauma injuries, beware of the high frequency of associated globe injuries with lid lacerations. Lid lacerations with canalicular involvement, lid-margin involvement, full-thickness penetration, loss of tissue, fat prolapse, or ptosis require definitive ophthalmic intervention and should be triaged immediately to an ophthalmologist. Other simple lid lacerations may be treated with suture repair, avoiding lid-margin retraction. Foreign bodies in the lid should be removed and tetanus prophylaxis provided, if indicated.

Corneal Abrasions and Foreign Bodies
Diagnosis of corneal abrasions is facilitated by use of topical fluorescein and illumination of the ocular surface with cobalt-blue-filtered light. Non-penetrating foreign bodies can be removed with loupe magnification.

Treatment
- Remove non-penetrating foreign bodies with a cotton-tip applicator. A clinician or practitioner can use a spud or needle if appropriate magnification is available.
- Apply a topical antibiotic drop or ointment.
- Apply patch or provide lid closure.
- Treat intense ultraviolet exposure as a corneal abrasion.
- Remove contact lenses if cornea is affected.

Red Eye

In a trauma setting, the most common cause of red eye is a benign condition called a *subjunctival hemorrhage*. Examination should be directed at ruling out more serious injury to the globe.

In the absence of trauma, a red eye will most commonly be caused by allergy, viral or bacterial infection, or intraocular inflammation. Evaluation should be directed at determining if corneal involvement is present. Corneal involvement (keratitis or corneal ulcer) is potentially serious and can be identified by direct inspection of the cornea.

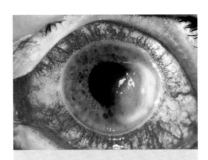

Figure 18.6
Red eye with corneal ulcer

Treatment

- Subconjunctival hemorrhages, without associated intraocular damage, do not require treatment.

- Red eyes with corneal involvement or decreased vision require more urgent ophthalmic evaluation and possible treatment.

- In the setting of biological or chemical terrorism/exposure, ophthalmic evaluation is required based on vision and corneal involvement.

Biological Agents and Eye Injuries

Botulism

Clinical Effects

- Cranial nerve dysfunction with ptosis, diplopia, and blurred vision followed by descending flaccid paralysis and respiratory insufficiency

- Eye signs usually bilateral

- Severity of *ophthalmoparesis* (weakness of the eye muscles) is a good indicator of overall severity of infection.

- Approximately 75% of patients with third-nerve palsy develop respiratory insufficiency.

Eye-Specific Treatment

- Provide supportive measures.

- Close one eye to eliminate diplopia.

Q Fever

Clinical Effects

- General flu symptoms with fever and headache, redness, conjunctival papillae, swelling, *petechiae* (tiny red spots), iritis, retinitis, and optic neuritis

Eye-Specific Treatment

- Provide artificial-tear supplementation for ocular surface irritation.
- Refer for ophthalmic evaluation to assess for intraocular inflammation.

Smallpox

Clinical Effects

- Fever, headache, maculopapular rash, severe prostration
- Nonspecific conjunctivitis
- Ocular surface pustule formation and hypopyon ulceration are more rare and severe.

Eye-Specific Treatment

- Provide artificial-tear lubrication to protect ocular surface.

Anthrax

While inhalation of *Bacillus anthracis* spores poses the potential for high mortality, cutaneous infection via direct contact with broken skin is rarely systemic. Eyes are spared by anthrax, but eyelids may be involved by direct skin contact.

Clinical Effects

- Eyelid discoloration, *maculae* (spots) leading to papule *vesiculation* (blistering), necrotic ulcer formation, and a black *eschar* (dry scab)

Eye-Specific Treatment

No eye treatment required. Utilize systemic antibiotic therapy if eyelid-skin involvement.

Ebola and Viral Hemorrhagic Fever

Clinical Effects

- Fever, headache, fatigue, and abdominal pain
- Nonspecific signs of conjunctivitis, uveitis, and very rarely, blindness

Eye-Specific Treatment

- Provide artificial-tear supplementation for ocular surface irritation.
- Refer to ophthalmologist for treatment of intraocular inflammation.

Tularemia—Parinaud's Oculoglandular Syndrome
Clinical Effects
- Flu symptoms with chest pain in inhalation-contracted disease

- With aerosol or direct eye contact, lid swelling, pre-auricular and cervical lymph node swelling, conjunctivitis with yellow-tinged ulcers and *chemosis* (conjunctival swelling)

Eye-Specific Treatment
- Provide artificial tear supplementation for ocular surface irritation.

Clostridium Tetanii
C.tetanii causes > one million cases/yr worldwide, mostly in developing countries without immunization programs. Infection follows contamination of wounds by soil or manure containing *C.tetanii*.

Clinical effects
- Spastic paralysis of muscles, including jaw muscles ("lock-jaw"), facial muscles ("sardonic smile"), back muscles (rigid, arched back) and respiratory muscles (respiratory failure).

- Cephalic tetanus (rare) can cause cranial-nerve palsies resulting in diplopia.

- Any trauma to the lids or eye, including lacerations, abrasions, intraocular foreign bodies, bites, and ruptured globes, can result in *C.tetanii* infection. The exception to this rule is that corneal abrasions alone (with no other associated trauma) are not at risk for causing tetanus.

Eye Specific treatment
- Tetanus immunization (tetanus toxoid or DPT) should be administered to injured patients who are: unimmunized, if tetanus immunization is >10 years old, or if immunization status is unknown.

- Tetanus immune globulin (TIG) should be administered if tetanus is suspected clinically.

Summary

Ocular injuries are common in all disasters regardless of etiology and present a challenge to medical providers. Life-saving interventions are always the first priority. However, following initial stabilization of the victim, it is important to recognize vision-threatening eye injuries to prevent long-term complications of blindness and cosmetic disfigurement.

KEY POINTS

 Copious irrigation with Normal Saline (NS) or water— <u>not</u> neutralization of the chemical agent—is the first priority in treating cases of chemical injuries to the eye.

 Triage personnel should have a high index of suspicion for globe rupture in all cases of orbital trauma.

 When treating eye injuries in a non-ophthalmologic setting, the use of NS rinses, topical antibiotic eye drops, and eye shields are the safest initial interventions.

Ear Injuries

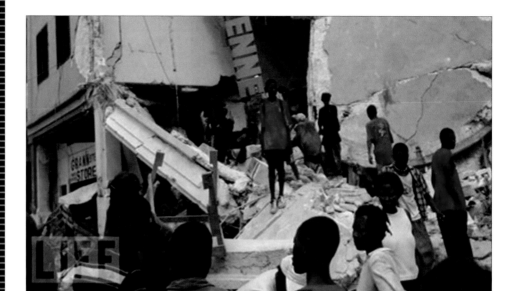

Fig.19.1 Haiti earthquake (2010)

CASE SCENARIO

A 32-year-old male was pulled from a collapsed building by search and rescue teams following the Haiti earthquake. He was brought to a field hospital with the history of being struck in the head by falling debris from a damaged structure. He complained of pain in the left side of the head, vertigo with nausea and vomiting worsened by head movement, and loss of hearing in the left ear. Vital signs were stable.

He had a spontaneous right-beating nystagmus, a simple helical laceration of his left auricle, and a small hematoma overlaying the left mastoid process. Examination of both ear canals and the right tympanic membrane were normal. However, his left tympanic membrane had an air-fluid level. There was no otorrhea. His hearing was normal to whispered speech on the right, reduced on the left. Tuning fork (512 Hz) test showed air conduction better than bone on the right, and bone better than air on the left. There was mild facial weakness in both the upper and lower divisions of the facial nerve on the left.

He was diagnosed with a labyrinthine concussion and a longitudinal fracture of the temporal bone involving the middle ear, with cerebrospinal fluid (CSF) in the middle ear. He was advised to have imaging studies when available. His laceration was sutured, and he was observed over the next two days with no change in his otoscopic exam, slight improvement in his nystagmus and vertigo, and gradual improvement of his facial paresis.

Introduction

Ear trauma is common in disasters, most often in conjunction with other traumatic injuries, and is often missed in the initial triage and evaluation of disaster victims. Ear trauma can also be a marker for more significant craniofacial trauma requiring immediate medical interventions.

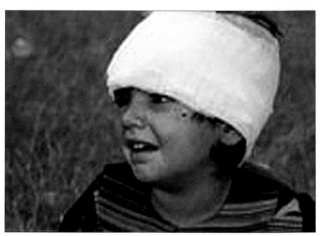

Fig.19.2 Child with blunt ear trauma

Otoscopic Evaluation

Is the canal intact?

The anterior canal wall is the posterior articular surface of the temporomandibular joint. Is there <u>pain</u> or <u>limitation</u> of occlusion? Fractures may be hidden by hematoma or bleeding into the canal. If the canal is clear, a <u>step- off</u> or bone <u>fragment</u> may be seen. If suction is unavailable, a Q-tip or drops may be used to remove blood from the lateral portion of the canal. There is no substitute for an otoscope if available.

Is the tympanic membrane (TM) intact?

If perforated, is there <u>leakage</u> of clear fluid (CSF) or blood? If intact, is there an <u>air-fluid level or a blue TM</u> indicative of CSF or blood in the middle ear.

Hearing Evaluation

Evaluation of hearing in the field can be done by whispering in the ear while masking the hearing in the contralateral ear by gently rubbing the auricle to make a sound louder than the whisper. A noise generator, such as an alarm clock, can be used to mask loud (even shouted) speech to evaluate for total hearing loss. If a loss is detected (e.g., cannot perceive whispered speech), a tuning fork test should be done to differentiate middle ear loss from inner ear loss. Inner ear loss when it occurs in trauma is almost always total. A 512 Hz fork is used, and air conduction (fork tines held within 2 inches of the auricle) is compared to the sound heard by placing the handle end of the fork on the mastoid process. Normally, the sound is louder when the fork is held next to the ear. Hearing the fork louder when vibrating the mastoid (i.e. bypassing the middle ear) indicates a conductive (middle ear pathology) loss.

> **TREATMENT ALERT!**
> **Tuning Fork Test**
>
> Air > Bone = normal or sensorineural loss
> Bone > Air = conductive hearing loss

Facial nerve evaluation

The trauma victim is first asked to smile to evaluate the lower division of Cranial Nerve VII (CN VII) and then to close his/her eyes tightly to evaluate the upper division. Right-left symmetry is judged as well as upper -lower equality of motion. Immediate-onset paralysis from trauma indicates an injury to the facial nerve in the region extending from the brain stem to the exit of the nerve from the skull in front of the mastoid. Both upper and lower divisions are usually affected. One division - only paralysis usually indicates a peripheral etiology distal to the exit from the mastoid.

Vestibular System Evaluation

The vestibular system can be evaluated by examining the eye motion, both spontaneously or provoked by position change. Rapid fast-slow motion of the eyes (nystagmus) can be vertical, horizontal, or rotatory. Vertical nystagmus is indicative of CNS injury, whereas horizontal and rotatory nystagmus indicates peripheral (labyrinthine) pathology.

External Ear Injuries

Attention is given to the <u>depth of lacerations in the auricle</u> as cartilage exposure risks infection, which frequently results in cartilage loss and subsequent deformity. **Judgment of cartilage exposure is important in the decision to institute antibiotic coverage.** <u>Devitalized skin (and cartilage)</u> should be generously debrided prior to skin closure. This need not be extensive in most cases as the ear is well-vascularized. A wedge excision of the auricle results in a smaller but cosmetically superior auricle.

Bleeding is a common problem because of the excellent blood supply of the ear. <u>Bleeding</u> can usually be controlled by pressure alone. Attention must be given to the presence of any <u>hematoma</u>. Blood collection in the subperichondrium may result in loss of cartilage and subsequent deformity. A very small hematoma (<1 cm.) may be observed and treated with a pressure dressing. A large hematoma requires drainage under sterile conditions and a conforming pressure dressing with both sides of the auricle being padded. Cotton impregnated with antibiotic ointment is used to make a conforming dressing. <u>Hematoma</u> overlying the mastoid prominence (Battle's sign) is indicative of a temporal bone fracture and disruption of the emissary veins from the sigmoid sinus. If the fracture extends to the periphery, a <u>step off</u> is palpable in the mastoid bone.

Canal injuries include <u>lacerations</u> for which topical antibiotic therapy (e.g. Ciprofloxacin drops) is indicated. Often fractures show a mixed pattern (i.e., longitudinal and transverse). <u>Foreign bodies</u> should be removed atraumatically, and post-removal topical antibiotics administered.

Middle Ear Injuries

Otoscopic examination of the TM can give valuable information. An air-fluid level behind the drum can indicate a CSF leak following a temporal bone fracture. In a blow to the ear, the TM may be ruptured. Also, direct trauma by a foreign body (e.g., Q-tip or welding spark) can perforate the TM.

Ossicular damage, when it occurs, is usually a dislocation of the malleus or incus with subsequent conductive hearing loss (Bone > Air). This can occur with blunt or sharp trauma as discussed above, which usually (not always) includes a rupture of the TM. Ossicular discontinuity also occurs with an intact TM after closed head trauma. No immediate therapy is required and the condition can be dealt with at a later date (reconstructive surgery for hearing restoration).

Inner Ear Injuries

The sensory organ of the ear is encased in bone, the otic capsule, imbedded in the petrous portion of the temporal bone, which forms the floor of the middle cranial fossa. The internal auditory canal, through which traverse the seventh and eighth nerves, is located in the medial part of the petrous portion of the temporal bone. Fractures of the temporal bone from blunt head trauma are either longitudinal, horizontal, or mixed. Longitudinal fractures, usually result from temporoparietal trauma, but also occur in fronto-occipital trauma. Although 20% of these fractures result in CN VII injury, most of the damage is in the middle ear and external auditory canal. Horizontal (transverse) temporal bone fractures usually result in deafness, vertigo as the fracture involves the otic capsule, and CN VII palsy. The external canal and middle ear are usually spared.

Temporal Bone Fractures

Longitudinal (80%)

- Temporoparietal trauma > fronto-occipital
- 20% have facial nerve injury
- Middle ear and canal injury most common

Horizontal (20%)

- Tympanic membrane intact
- Sensorineural hearing loss
- Vertigo
- CN VII palsy (50%)

Temporal bone fracture should be suspected in any patient who has received significant blunt trauma to the head. Temporo-parietal trauma is the more common traumatic injury in longitudinal, middle cranial fossa fractures. **Red flags for these injuries are hearing loss and vertigo (VIII CN), facial paresis (VII CN), a mastoid process hematoma (Battle's sign) and bloody (or clear CSF) otorrhea.** Horizontal temporal bone (floor of middle cranial fossa) fractures usually occur with trauma of greater force. Often, the fracture extends into the occipital bone, in which case the brain stem is involved, and the condition is usually incompatible with life (the coroner's fracture). Horizontal bone fractures may cause CN VII and VIII injuries, the red flags being vertigo, hearing loss, and facial paresis.

Cranial Nerve (CN) VII Injury

Immediate onset

- Transection or severe damage by bone fragments
- Consider immediate surgery if patient is neurologically stable.

Delayed onset (hours)

- Caused by edema
- One third resolve spontaneously
- Consider steroid therapy

Facial nerve injury from temporal bone fractures results in weakness or total paralysis of facial motion. In trauma, it is unlikely, but not impossible, to see facial nerve injury in the absence of a fracture. The treatment options are the same: surgical decompression of the bony facial nerve canal for total paralysis or observation with steroids for partial paralysis, with consideration for decompression therapy if the paralysis becomes total. It is the edema about the nerve in the canal that compromises blood flow, ultimately leading to death of the nerve which is the basis for decompression surgery. These observations are important in triage and initial evaluation of patients with facial trauma, as this directly affects the ultimate outcome in terms of facial animation.

Summary

Ear trauma, although usually not life-threatening, can lead to significant morbidity and cosmetic deformities if injuries are missed. Otoscopic evaluation is a valuable asset in the initial evaluation.

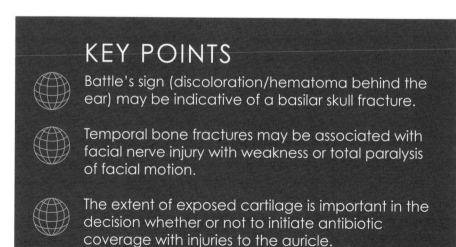

KEY POINTS

- Battle's sign (discoloration/hematoma behind the ear) may be indicative of a basilar skull fracture.

- Temporal bone fractures may be associated with facial nerve injury with weakness or total paralysis of facial motion.

- The extent of exposed cartilage is important in the decision whether or not to initiate antibiotic coverage with injuries to the auricle.

Burn Injuries

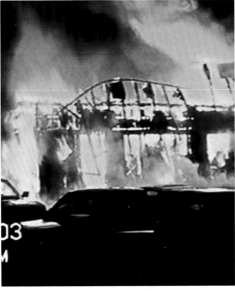 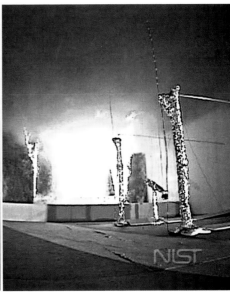

Fig.20.1 Rhode Island nightclub fire, Courtesy of Rhode Island Attorney General

Fig.20.2 Simulation of Rhode Island nightclub fire, Courtesy of NIST.gov

CASE SCENARIO

The Station nightclub fire, which occurred in Rhode Island on February 20, 2003, was one of the deadliest nightclub fires in the United States. The fast-moving fire was caused by pyrotechnics used in conjunction with the band's performance that evening. Approximately 100 individuals were killed and 200 victims injured.

Introduction

Burn injuries are common in disasters. There are several types of burns seen in these settings: scald, flame, chemical, electrical, and radiation. Although treatment protocols vary for different types and degrees of burns, the first priorities in the care of a burn patient at a disaster scene are to stop the burning process and manage associated injuries. Blast and crush injuries are common in burn patients.

Classification of Burn Injuries

Burns may be classified into four degrees, depending upon the severity of damage, as described below.

- **First-Degree Burns (Partial Thickness)**

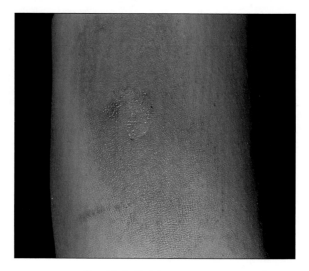

Fig. 20.3 First-Degree Burn
Symptoms: redness; pain
Treatment: topical agents for pain

First-degree burns involve only the epidermis and are characterized by cutaneous erythema and mild pain. Tissue damage is minimal. Pain, the chief symptom, usually resolves in 48–72 hours. Overexposure to sunlight and brief scalding by hot liquids are the most common causes of first-degree burns.

- ## Second-Degree Burns (Partial Thickness)

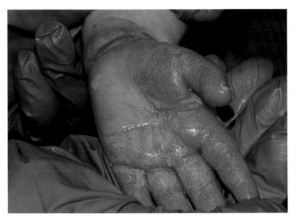

Fig. 20.4 Second-Degree Burn
Symptoms: vesicle (blister) formation; pain
Treatment: topical agents for pain; skin grafting

Second-degree burns involve injury to the entire epidermis and variable portions of the dermal layer. *Vesicle* (blister) formation and pain are characteristic. Deeper second-degree burns can be less painful.

- ## Third-Degree Burns (Full Thickness)

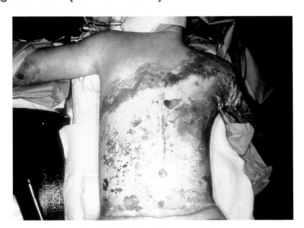

Fig. 20.5 Third-Degree Burn
Symptoms: leathery, dry, usually painless
Treatment: skin grafting; small third-degree
burns may heal by 2° contraction

Third-degree burns, or full-thickness burns, involve the destruction of the entire epidermis and dermis, leaving no cells to regenerate skin. Third-degree burns are relatively painless due to heat destruction of nerve endings.

- **Fourth-Degree Burns**

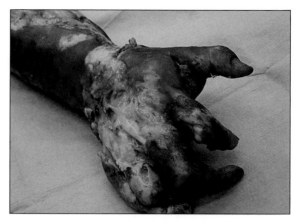

Fig. 20.6 Fourth-Degree Burn
Symptoms: deep charring of underlying tendons,
muscle, bone
Treatment: wound management is complex

Fourth-degree burns destroy the dermis and damage the underlying tendons, muscle, and bone. Wound management of these burns is complex and always requires triage to a hospital for definitive medical care.

Emergency Management of Burns

Patients with serious burn injuries are similar to other trauma patients. Initial evaluation and management should assume coincident trauma. Associated non-burn injuries will make resuscitation needs unpredictable.

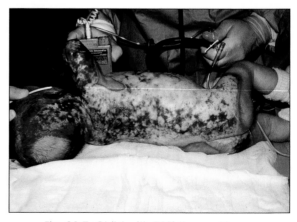

Fig. 20.7 Child with 70% thermal burns

Airway Management

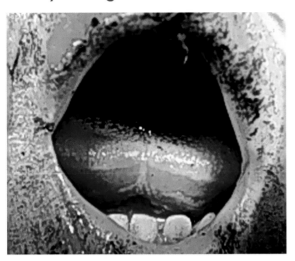

Fig. 20.8 Inhalation Injury

- Ensure patency of airway (with C-spine control).

- Indications for intubation are:

    o Massive facial swelling

    o Inhalation injury

- Administer oxygen via face mask or endotracheal tube. Maintain breathing and circulation as needed.

- Evaluate for smoke inhalation injury. **Symptoms of smoke inhalation include hypoxia (low O_2), hypercapnia (high CO_2), and carbon monoxide poisoning.** Inhalation injury is often a cause of early death in burns and can be a more important determinant of survival than burn size.

FIELD OBSERVATION

Signs suspicious for inhalation injury include:

- **Upper body burns**
- **Singeing of eyebrows and nasal hair**
- **Soot in oropharynx**
- **History of impaired mental activity and/or confinement in a burning environment (closed-space injury)**
- **Carbonaceous sputum (soot-like material)**

Fluid Resuscitation

Commence fluid resuscitation using isotonic electrolyte solutions such as Ringer's Lactate.

- **Calculation of fluid requirements for resuscitation is based on an estimate of second-degree and third-degree burns only.**

- Fluid resuscitation is calculated via formulae such as the modified Parkland Fluid Resuscitation Formula.

- Percentage of burn is calculated using the "Rule of Nines."

- **Time of burn injury is starting point for 24 hours—not time of treatment initiation.**

DETERMINING BURN SIZE

An estimate of burn size is important in calculating fluid resuscitation.

- **Use the "Rule of Nines" to estimate burn size.**

- **For areas of irregular or nonconfluent area burns, use the palmar surface of the patient's hand, which represents approximately 1% of the body surface.**

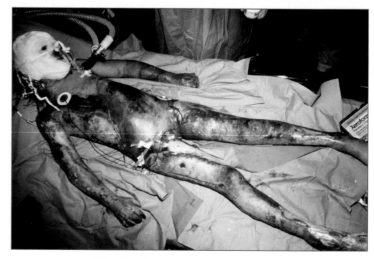

Fig. 20.9 Severe thermal burn injury

Standard of Practice: Rule of Nines
Note: Children have significantly larger heads and smaller legs than adults.

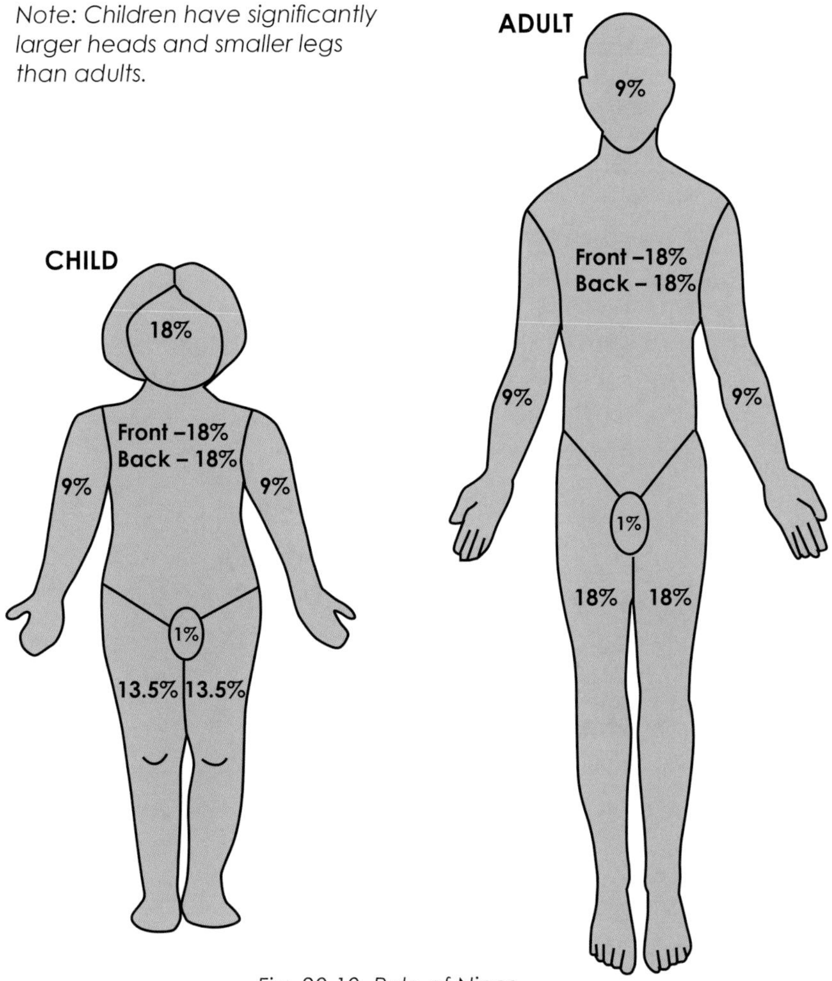

Fig. 20.10 Rule of Nines

MODIFIED PARKLAND FLUID RESUSCITATION FORMULA

**Fluids for first 24 hours = 4 cc x kg x % burn
(second-degree and third-degree burns only)**

o First-half of fluid requirement in the first 8 hours
o Second-half of fluid requirement over the following 16 hours
o Measured from time of burn, not time of treatment initiation
o Ringer's Lactate (RL) fluid of choice
o Titrate RL to urine output with 0.5–1.0 cc/kg/hr target

Secondary Priorities in Burn Management

After stabilizing the patient:

- Perform a detailed head-to-toe examination. Assume other injuries are likely to be present in disaster scenarios.

- Delayed resuscitation is common in disaster scenarios.

- Obtain history from witnesses, rescue personnel, or family members.

  o Mechanism of injury will dictate need for other tests.

  o Age, weight, past medical and surgical history, time of last meal, tetanus status, and history of "closed-space environment" are all-important factors in the treatment of burn victims.

- Treat associated injuries.

- Administer tetanus toxoid (0.5 cc sc) if no booster in last 5 years, or if date of last booster is unknown.

- For individuals not immunized against tetanus, administer 250 units of human tetanus immunoglobulin.

- **Antibiotics are generally not used prophylactically.**

- Most casualties with burns > 20% of body surface develop a reflex paralytic ileus during the first 24 hours, which may require nasogastric decompression.

- Full-thickness burns of thorax and extremities (including digits) may cause constriction of underlying structures. A constricting *eschar* (full-thickness burn) of the thorax may result in life-threatening respiratory depression and may mandate immediate escharotomy. **An *escharotomy* is a linear incision extending through the full depth of the burned skin, allowing separation of the full-thickness burn.**

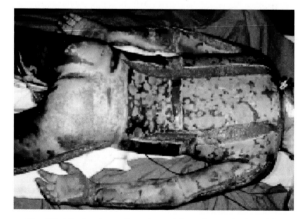

Fig.20.11 Escharotomies of back and chest in child with 70% thermal burns.

230

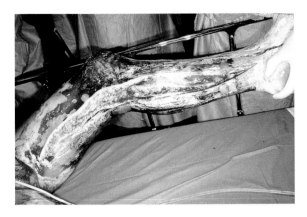

Fig. 20.12 Escharotomy of lower extremity in patient with thermal burns secondary to motor vehicle accident.

Chemical Burns

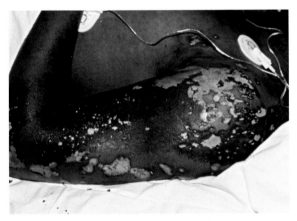

Fig. 20.13 Sulfuric acid chemical burn

While chemical burns present many of the same issues as other thermal burns, there are special considerations that apply. **Self-protection is critical when decontaminating wounds!**

- Medical responders must be careful to protect themselves from secondary chemical exposure.

- Remove casualty's clothing as quickly as possible to minimize damage caused by absorbed chemical agents.

- Remove viscous liquids mechanically (e.g., by scraping with a tongue depressor or stick).

- **Break blisters to stop the burning process—blisters often contain the chemical agent.**

- Copiously irrigate affected areas with water, including eyes.

TREATMENT ALERT!

In chemical burns, blisters often contain the burning agent and should be broken and irrigated to stop the burning process.

231

- After thorough skin decontamination, cover burn with clean, dry sheets.
- **The concentration of the chemical agent and the duration of exposure are key factors in determining the extent of thermal injury.**

Special Considerations in Chemical Burns

Several chemical compounds present special problems in burn casualties. Four of these – white phosphorous, cement, tar, and hydrofluoric acid – are discussed here.

White Phosphorus

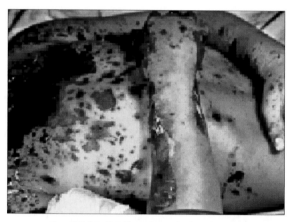

Fig. 20.14 White phosphorus burns

- Particulate solid that may ignite spontaneously in air at 34°C (93.2°F)
- Military and civilian uses, including agent found in munitions, fertilizers, insecticides, and fireworks
- Treat with copious amounts of **COLD** water – avoid warm water as white phosphorous becomes liquid at 44°C (111.2°F).
- Cover imbedded particles with cool saline dressings to prevent ignition before surgical removal.

Cement

- Contains lime (calcium oxide).
- Forms calcium hydroxide when mixed with water – perspiration is sufficient to support this reaction.
- May cause alkali burns to skin and eyes.
- Flush with large amounts of water.

Tar

- Generally heated to 149°– 260°C (300°–500°F)
- Initial cooling with copious irrigation with cool water
- Subsequent removal with lipophyllic solvents (butter, baby oil, sunflower oil, etc.)

Hydrofluoric Acid (HFA)

- Used as rust remover and cleaner, as well as in glass and silicon etching, plastics manufacture, and semiconductor fabrication
- Dilute vs. concentrated forms
- **Dilute HFA**
    - o Exposure results in delayed symptoms.
    - o Topical treatments for exposure to dilute HFA include calcium gluconate (2.5% gel), magnesium oxide ointment, ammonium compounds (Hibiclens or Zephiran).
- **Concentrated HFA**
    - o Exposure brings risk of cardiac arrhythmias due to hypocalcemia and hypomagnesemia.
    - o Risk of respiratory failure
    - o Risk of sudden death
    - o Irrigation and subeschar injection with 10% calcium gluconate until pain resolution
    - o Beware of inhalation of vapors with subsequent bronchospasm and respiratory failure

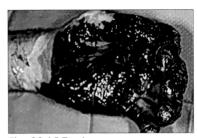

Fig. 20.15 Tar burn

Treatment Tip

Maalox or calcium gluconate can be mixed with Surgilube® or KY jelly® to form a topical treatment for dilute HFA burns.

Electrical Burns

Electrical burns require special attention at the disaster scene. Various factors influence the degree of tissue damage in electrical burns, including type and voltage of the current, resistance, pathway of transmission in the body, and duration of contact.

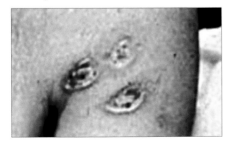

*Fig. 20.16 Arc electrical injury,
Courtesy of NIST.gov*

The first task is for the rescue team to remove the casualty from the source of the electrical current <u>without</u> becoming a part of the electrical circuit themselves!

Several types of injury occur in electrical accidents:

- <u>Deep conductive electrical injuries</u> involve extensive muscle damage, the extent of which may not be obvious at the scene.
- <u>Arc injuries</u> produce limited, deep areas of coagulation damage, especially in flexion areas such as axilla or groin.
- <u>Surface thermal burns</u> occur as the result of flash ignition of clothing and must be treated with stoppage of the burning process (e.g., removal of burning clothing).
- <u>Electrical burn-injury casualties</u> often present with total surface area (TSA) thermal burns.
- <u>Associated trauma</u>, often related to falls, is common. Look for:
    - o Head injuries
    - o Cervical spine injuries
    - o Long bones fractures
    - o Thoracoabdominal injuries
- <u>Cardiac arrhythmias</u>, including asystole and ventricular fibrillation, are common in electrical burn casualties.
- <u>Compartment syndromes</u> in upper and lower extremities are common in electrical injuries as well. Severe muscle damage results in *myoglobinuria* (myoglobin in the urine), which usually manifests as dark urine.

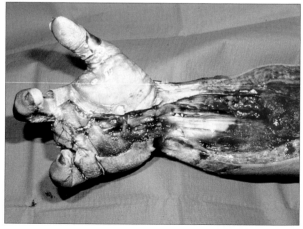

Fig. 20.17 Upper extremity and hand fasciotomies in patient with compartment syndrome secondary to electrical injury.

Summary

Burn injuries are common in both natural and man-made disasters and often accompanied by associated traumatic injuries. **The first priority in the care of all burn victims is to "stop the burning process."** Chemical and electrical injuries present complex challenges in care for medical providers.

KEY POINTS

Calculation of the fluid requirement for resuscitation of burn victims is based <u>on second-degree and third-degree burns only</u> (first-degree burns not included in burn resuscitation formula).

Massive facial swelling and inhalation injury are leading causes for intubation of burn victims.

<u>Copious irrigation</u> of the affected areas is a key priority in the initial management of chemical burns.

The first priority in electrical burns is to remove the casualty from the source of the electrical current <u>without</u> becoming a part of the electrical circuit.

Altitude Illnesses

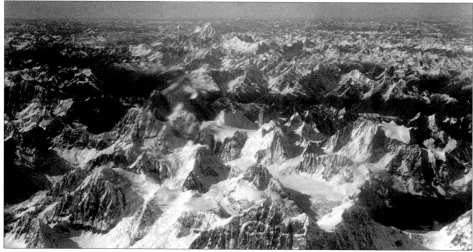

Fig. 21.1 Tibet, China

CASE SCENARIO

An avalanche strikes a remote ski hut at 3400m. One of the wounded occupants radios for help, and a rescue team is dispatched by helicopter from the nearest town (elevation 1000m). The rescuers have no time to acclimatize to high altitude and begin working strenuously to extricate victims immediately upon arrival. The following day, several of the rescuers are suffering from headache and lethargy, but bad weather prevents helicopter evacuation. They refuse to descend, insisting that they are fine and must continue to aid the avalanche victims. After the second night, one rescuer is severely short of breath with minimal exertion and cyanotic. His HR=120, and O_2 Sat=66%. He is diagnosed with HAPE. Nifedipine, oxygen, and bed rest are administered, and he stabilizes until the weather clears and evacuation can be arranged.

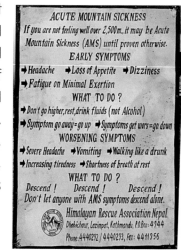

Fig. 21.2 Warning sign posted by Himalayan Rescue Association (Nepal)

Introduction

Disaster responders may sometimes be required to work in a high-altitude environment or to treat victims of altitude illness. Beyond the usual medical consequences of a natural or man-made disaster, when such an event occurs above an altitude of 2500m (approximately 8200ft), hypobaria (decreased barometric pressure) and its attendant hypoxia (low O_2) introduce additional physiological stresses and considerations for both disaster victims and rescuers.

Hypobaric hypoxia is the most important environmental factor associated with ascent to altitude and is the underlying cause of clinical altitude illness. As barometric pressure decreases with increasing altitude, the partial pressure of inspired oxygen (PIO_2) progressively falls. A number of mechanisms, collectively known as acclimatization, allow people to adjust to the hypoxic environment of high altitude. However, acclimatization takes time, and, when one ascends faster than one can acclimatize, clinical altitude illness results.

Prevention

Factors impacting the risk of altitude illness include:

- **Elevation** – the higher the elevation, the greater the risk

- **Rate of ascent** – the faster the ascent, the greater the risk

- **Exertion** – strenuous exercise is a risk factor

- **Individual susceptibility** – a history of altitude-related illness is a risk factor for developing recurrent disease.

The best way to manage altitude illness is to prevent it.

Current recommendations include the following:

- Do not ascend directly from low altitude to higher than 2500m.

- Above 2500m, do not increase sleeping altitude by more than 300-500m/night, and take a rest day (do not ascend at all) every 2-3 days.

- If gradual ascent is not possible, take acetazolamide 125-250mg by mouth twice daily for prophylaxis. Start 24 hours before ascent and continue for 2-3 days after maximum altitude is reached.

- For rescue teams that must travel to very high altitude (>3500m) without acclimatizing, dexamethasone 4mg by mouth every six hours can be used for prophylaxis.

TREATMENT ALERT!

Gradual ascent is the best way to prevent altitude illness. If not possible, take acetazolamide 125-250 mg PO BID. Acetazolamide produces a mild metabolic acidosis that enhances ventilation (respiratory stimulant effect) and reduces hypoxemia.

Acute Mountain Sickness (AMS)

Acute mountain sickness (AMS) is the most common high-altitude syndrome. How exactly hypoxia causes the syndrome is unknown, but it is likely that increased cerebral blood flow, vasogenic cerebral edema, and possibly increased intracranial pressure play important roles.

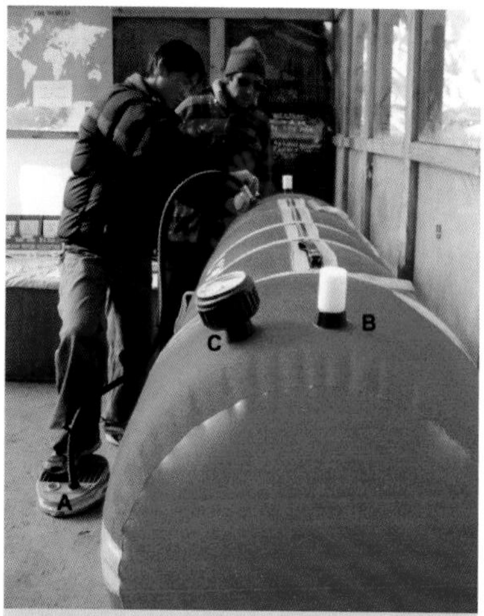

Clinical Characteristics

Acute mountain sickness typically manifests 4-6 hours or more after an increase in altitude. The diagnosis is based on the presence of headache, and at least one of the following symptoms:

- Gastrointestinal symptoms: anorexia, nausea, vomiting
- Fatigue/weakness
- Lassitude, apathy, irritability
- Dizziness and light-headedness
- Insomnia

While mild exertional dyspnea is normal and to be expected at high altitude, severe dyspnea or dyspnea at rest heralds the onset of high-altitude pulmonary edema (HAPE). Similarly, altered mental status and ataxia are the clinical hallmarks of high-altitude cerebral edema (HACE). These are the most serious forms of acute altitude illness and often preceded by AMS.

Treatment

- **Stop ascending.** If symptoms are severe (severe headache, repeated vomiting, symptoms not relieved with over-the-counter analgesics), consider descending to a lower altitude; 500 to 1,000m is usually adequate to relieve symptoms.
- Headache can be treated with ibuprofen (400-600mg every 6 hours) and nausea with antiemetics (compazine 10mg by mouth).
- Administer acetazolamide (125 to 250mg twice daily by mouth).
- Allow the patient to rest.
- Administer oxygen (1-3 L/min will usually suffice).
- If oxygen supplies are limited and descent is not possible, a portable hyperbaric chamber (e.g., Gamow bag or portable altitude chamber) is effective.
- Administer dexamethasone (4mg by mouth or intramuscularly every 6 hours) for moderate to severe AMS if the other therapies listed above are not effective.

Fig. 21.3
The Gamow bag is a portable hyperbaric chamber. The patient is inserted into the bag, and the zipper is closed. The foot pump (A) generates pressure and circulates air through the bag. The pressure valve (B) allows air to escape when a pressure of 2 pounds per square inch is reached. The pressure gauge (C) monitors pressure in the chamber.

FIELD OBSERVATION

Acute Mountain Sickness (AMS) is the most common high-altitude syndrome.

High-Altitude Pulmonary Edema (HAPE)

A more serious potential consequence of exposure to high altitude is high-altitude pulmonary edema (HAPE). **HAPE is a form of noncardiogenic pulmonary edema.** It occurs when hypoxia induces pulmonary vasoconstriction leading to pulmonary hypertension. This causes the normally low-pressure pulmonary vasculature to break down, resulting in fluid leak into the alveoli. HAPE is the most common cause of death due to altitude illness.

Clinical Characteristics

Symptoms usually begin 24-72 hours after ascent. At least half the time HAPE is preceded or accompanied by symptoms of AMS. Severe dyspnea with exertion that progresses to dyspnea at rest is the most prominent symptom. Cough, chest tightness, and severe fatigue or weakness are also common. **The predominance of respiratory symptoms (dyspnea at rest) allows HAPE to be clinically distinguished from AMS.**

Physical exam reveals tachypnea, tachycardia, and possibly low-grade fever. Hypoxemia is often severe. The victim will have pulmonary crackles, which may even be audible without a stethoscope and may be unilateral or bilateral. Cyanosis develops as the disease progresses. HAPE patients may initially appear well, but once the stage of dyspnea at rest is reached, can progress to death within a few hours if untreated.

Treatment

- Rapidly descend to lower altitude.
- Administer supplemental oxygen at 4 to 6 L/min to immediately reduce pulmonary hypertension, which rapidly alleviates dyspnea and tachycardia.
- If oxygen supplies are limited and descent is not possible, a portable hyperbaric chamber may be a useful temporizing measure.
- Allow the patient to rest, since exercise exacerbates pulmonary hypertension.
- Keep the patient warm, since cold stress can elevate pulmonary arterial pressure.
- While drug therapy is less valuable than descent or supplemental oxygen, nifedipine is effective (10mg immediate release, followed by 30mg, sustained release by mouth every 12 hours).
- A number of drugs, including inhaled salmeterol, dexamethasone, tadalafil, and sildenafil, appear to provide effective prophylaxis for individuals with a prior history of HAPE who are ascending to a high altitude. Their effectiveness for treatment has not been tested.

FIELD OBSERVATION

HAPE is the leading cause of death from altitude illness.

FIELD OBSERVATION

Successful treatment of HAPE depends on its early recognition. As with other altitude illnesses, descent to lower altitude is the mainstay of treatment.

239

High-Altitude Cerebral Edema (HACE)

High-altitude cerebral edema (HACE) is a serious neurological consequence of altitude exposure and can be thought of as the extreme form of acute mountain sickness (AMS).

Clinical Characteristics

Gait ataxia, mental status changes, and profound lassitude are the hallmarks of HACE. Headache and nausea are typical, and the victim may experience neurological manifestations, including hallucinations, cranial nerve palsy, hemiparesis, seizures, and focal neurological signs.

A rapid progression from confusion to stupor or coma may occur. The victim is often ashen or cyanotic, as well as profoundly hypoxic. Funduscopic exam may show papilledema. Coexistent pulmonary edema (HAPE) is common.

Treatment

- Rapidly descend to a lower altitude.
- Administer supplemental oxygen at 4-6 L/min.
- Administer dexamethasone promptly (8mg loading dose, followed by 4mg intravenously, intramuscularly, or orally every 6 hours).
- If HACE symptoms have been of long duration, the response to therapy may be slow. Additional supportive care, possibly including endotracheal intubation, should be implemented as needed depending on the response to the therapies listed above.

Other High-Altitude Medical Phenomena

Ultraviolet Keratitis

- Ultraviolet keratitis (snow blindness), the most common cause of radiation injury to the eye, occurs when the cornea is pathologically overexposed to ultraviolet (UV) sunlight.
- Ultraviolet radiation significantly increases with altitude, and the effect is magnified further by reflected UV radiation from snowfields.
- The condition presents with bilateral ocular pain, photosensitivity, conjunctival redness, and edema. It can be debilitating and render a victim effectively blind for >24 hours.
- In addition to cold compresses over the eyes, treatment involves topical anesthetics (e.g., tetracaine), systemic analgesics (opiates), anti-inflammatories (ibuprofen), and eye patching for at least 12 hours.
- Ultraviolet keratitis can be prevented by the use of appropriate eye protection, namely sunglasses or goggles with UV-A and UV-B protection with appropriate shields to prevent reflected light from entering around the lenses.

240

High-Altitude Retinopathy

- High altitude retinopathy refers to the frequent finding of retinal hemorrhages in travelers at high altitude.

- Usually asymptomatic and requires no treatment.

- Very rarely, if a retinal hemorrhage involves the macula, it may result in painless monocular blindness. This typically resolves with time.

High-Altitude Cough

- High altitude is associated with persistent cough in many individuals, which is sometimes productive of sputum and is occasionally vigorous enough to fracture ribs.

- There is no dyspnea at rest and oxygen saturation is normal for altitude.

- This may be due to increased ventilation, centrally mediated decrease in cough threshold, or other mechanisms.

- Once HAPE and pulmonary infection are ruled out, treatment is symptomatic, but often ineffective.

High-Altitude Peripheral Edema

- Occurs in 10-20% of people, more common in females. Most common in face, hands, and feet.

- Not associated with altitude illness.

- No treatment is necessary unless symptoms are bothersome. Can use acetazolamide or low-dose furosemide.

Planning for Disasters at Altitude

Those planning disaster responses at high altitude must pay attention to the following considerations:

Special drugs:

- Acetazolamide for the prevention and treatment of AMS

- Nifedipine for the treatment of HAPE

- Dexamethasone for the prevention and treatment of severe AMS and HACE.

Sources of oxygen:

- Oxygen may be needed to treat rescuers as well as victims of the disaster.

- Tanks are convenient and easily moved with individual patients but provide a finite supply, which must be constantly replaced.

- Oxygen concentrators provide a continuous source of oxygen, but require a source of electricity.

241

- A portable hyperbaric chamber (e.g., Gamow bag or PAC) is inexhaustible and does not require power. Disadvantages are that patients are difficult to move while in the chamber, there is no immediate access to a patient in the chamber, and another person is required to circulate air through the chamber. This method of treatment may only be justified for larger operations.

Transport

Helicopters do not function at their full capacity at high altitude since their rotors generate less lift in the thin air. Flying may be limited to good-weather conditions, loads may need to be lightened, and aircraft may need to be modified. This can substantially impact the logistics of disaster response, especially at very high altitudes.

Summary

It is likely that most disaster scenarios will occur at the customary altitudes of our urban population centers. But the possibility remains that such an event could transpire in a location where hypobaric hypoxia is the norm. In that case, medical responders will need to remain cognizant of the added physical and pathophysiological challenges of the high-altitude environment, both for their patients and themselves.

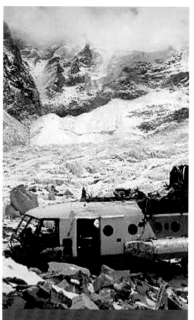

Fig. 21.4
Helicopter travel at high altitudes can be hazardous, as rotors generate less lift in the thin air. Shown here is wreckage of a helicopter at Mt. Everest basecamp (elevation 5380m).

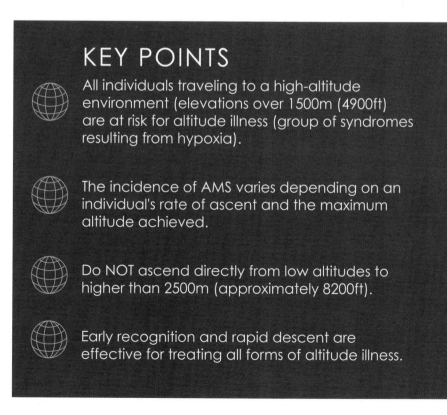

KEY POINTS

All individuals traveling to a high-altitude environment (elevations over 1500m (4900ft) are at risk for altitude illness (group of syndromes resulting from hypoxia).

The incidence of AMS varies depending on an individual's rate of ascent and the maximum altitude achieved.

Do NOT ascend directly from low altitudes to higher than 2500m (approximately 8200ft).

Early recognition and rapid descent are effective for treating all forms of altitude illness.

Heat Illnesses

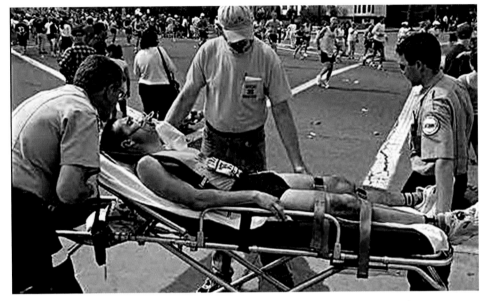

Fig. 22.1 *Boston Marathon runner with heat syncope (2012)*

CASE SCENARIO

The Boston Marathon, begun in 1897, is the world's oldest annual marathon and is known as one of the world's most prestigious road running events. The Marathon, 26 miles, 385 yards (42.195 kilometers) attracts over 20,000 runners and is always held on the third Monday in April. Heat-related injuries are a common condition requiring medical attention during this event. In 2012, with temperatures of 30°+C (high 80° F), over 2000 participants required medical attention, most for heat-related conditions.

Introduction

Heat-related illnesses are a continuum of physiologic disorders that, at their worst, result in an increase in body core temperature to levels that interfere with normal body functions and thermoregulation. Although they are described as discrete entities below, symptoms often overlap.

Environmental factors that influence exertional heat illnesses include:

- Ambient air temperature
- Peak temperature of the previous day
- Air relative humidity
- Wind velocity
- Mean radiant temperature
- Metabolic heat produced by the body

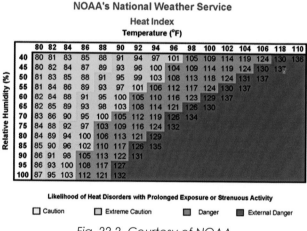

NOAA's National Weather Service
Heat Index
Temperature (°F)

Relative Humidity (%)	80	82	84	86	88	90	92	94	96	98	100	102	104	106	118	110
40	80	81	83	85	88	91	94	97	101	105	109	114	119	124	130	136
45	80	82	84	87	89	93	96	100	104	109	114	119	124	130	137	
50	81	83	85	88	91	95	99	103	108	113	118	124	131	137		
55	81	84	86	89	93	97	101	106	112	117	124	130	137			
60	82	84	88	91	95	100	105	110	116	123	129	137				
65	82	85	89	93	98	103	108	114	121	126	130					
70	83	86	90	95	100	105	112	119	126	134						
75	84	88	92	97	103	109	116	124	132							
80	84	89	94	100	106	113	121	129								
85	85	90	96	102	110	117	126	135								
90	86	91	98	105	113	122	131									
95	86	93	100	108	117	127										
100	87	95	103	112	121	132										

Likelihood of Heat Disorders with Prolonged Exposure or Strenuous Activity

☐ Caution   ☐ Extreme Caution   ☐ Danger   ■ External Danger

Fig. 22.2 Courtesy of NOAA

Personal factors that influence exertional heat illnesses include:

- Physical fitness and acclimatization
- Previous history of heat injury
- Obesity
- Age
- Fatigue
- Water consumption
- Alcohol consumption
- Work load
- Work habits

- Clothing worn
- Large skin abnormalities
    - o Burns
    - o Radiation scars
    - o Ectodermal dysplasia
- Medications
    - o Anticholinergics
    - o Antiepileptics
    - o Antihistamines
    - o Decongestants
    - o Tricyclic antidepressants
    - o Diuretics
    - o Beta blockers

Heat-Related Conditions

Heat Edema

Symptoms of heat edema include transient swelling of hands, ankles, and feet during the first few days of heat exposure from water retention and peripheral vasodilatation. The condition usually resolves after several days when the individual becomes acclimated. The body core temperature remains normal. Use of compression stockings and elevating the extremities when at rest in a cooler environment can reduce the swelling. Do not administer diuretics.

Heat Rash (Prickly Heat, Miliaria)

Blocked sweat ducts can produce acute inflammation and a maculopapular or vesicular rash, frequently affecting areas covered by tight clothing. Wearing light, loose-fitting clothing can help prevent its development. Treat the rash with chlorhexidine lotion to remove any desquamated skin. Treat the pruritus with topical or systemic antihistamines.

Heat Syncope

Intense sweating results in dehydration, peripheral vasodilatation, and postural hypotension.

- Also known as exercise-associated collapse. In an exercising individual, heat syncope usually occurs upon cessation of intense activity, resulting in a sudden decrease in venous return.

245

- In a non-exercising individual, heat syncope can occur after prolonged standing with little movement or with a sudden move to standing from a sitting or supine position.

- The body core temperature remains normal, and the mental status returns quickly to normal once the individual is supine.

- Treatment involves cooling, resting supine, and rehydration with either an oral rehydration solution or intravenous (IV) Normal Saline.

- Preventive measures include support stockings, deep knee-bending movements, and avoiding prolonged standing in the heat.

Heat Cramps

Also known as exercise-associated muscle cramps, characteristic symptoms are painful, involuntary spasms of large muscle groups used in strenuous exercise. Heat cramps tend to occur in individuals after intense exertion. Core temperature may be elevated, but < 40°C (104°F). The condition usually occurs when individuals are sweating profusely and replenish fluids with only non-electrolyte-containing water, resulting in hypochloremic hyponatremia.

- Mild: treat with oral 0.2% salt solutions

- Severe: IV isotonic fluids

- Sports drinks helpful

- Passively stretch involved muscles

- Avoid salt tablets. Frequently, there is inadequate fluid volume replacement while ingesting the tablets, and they can be gastric irritants causing nausea and vomiting.

Heat Tetany

Heat stress induces hyperventilation. Resulting respiratory alkalosis can cause severe carpopedal spasm, paresthesias, and tetany. Core temperature may be elevated, but < 40°C (104°F). Symptoms will resolve once the individual is removed from the hot environment and the respiratory rate decreases.

Heat Exhaustion

Heat exhaustion is typically associated with minor elevation of core temperature to < 40°C (104°F). It is not usually associated with evidence of organ damage or dysfunction, but delayed muscle necrosis may occur. Symptoms are quite varied and rapidly improve with water, salt replacement, and rest. Symptoms may include:

- Headache and light-headedness

- Tachycardia

- Hypotension

- Nausea, vomiting, and diarrhea

- Abdominal and muscle cramps

- Extreme weakness and syncope

Heat exhaustion most often comprises both water and salt depletion. The most common symptoms are excessive thirst, nausea, and muscle cramps. Treatment is focused on providing free water replacement and salt to casualties.

- In heat exhaustion from predominantly water depletion (usually from limited water supplies with high salt intake), symptoms are thirst, nausea, and muscle fatigue.

- In heat exhaustion from predominantly salt depletion (usually from limited salt supplies with high water intake), there are usually generalized muscle cramps. Individual patients can have highly variable salt-replacement needs. Salt loss can also be directly related to the amount of sweat produced and the salt content of that sweat.

Treatment of heat exhaustion includes:

- Stop exertion

- Move casualty to shaded, cool environment

- Remove victim's clothing down to underwear

- Controlled rehydration

- 0.5% oral saline solution (1 tsp salt/qt of water) or salty foods

- IV Normal Saline or Ringer's Lactate if unable to take fluids orally

Heat Injury

Defined by military physicians, heat injury describes those individuals with hyperthermia and end-organ damage, but without central nervous system (CNS) disturbances. Core temperatures are usually >104-105°F (40-40.5°C) and end-organ damage may include rhabdomyolysis, renal injury, and liver failure. Treatment is the same as for heat stroke (below).

Heat Stroke

Heat stroke is a **life-threatening** multi-system disorder reflecting collapse of the thermoregulatory system, a systemic inflammatory response, acid-base and electrolyte abnormalities, acute renal failure, muscle necrosis, and disseminated intravascular coagulation (DIC).

The hallmarks of heat stroke are a core temperature > 40°C (104°F) and CNS disturbances that can include headache, disorientation, confusion, seizures, and coma.

Heat Stroke

Classic	Exertional
Very young, elderly, chronically ill & socially isolated	Healthy young individuals
During heat waves – high temperatures & humidity	During heavy exertion and overwhelmed by metabolic heat production
Sweating absent in > 80%	Marked sweating
Frequently taking medications that interfere with heat loss	Hypoglycemia is common

Heat stroke is a medical emergency—mortality can reach 75% if left untreated. Long-term survival is directly related to the rapidity of resuscitative measures. Cooling should be immediately initiated. The degree of organ damage appears to be related to the magnitude of an individual's duration of elevated core temperature. Patients who cool slowly tend to have a more serious illness.

Treatment of Heat Stroke

<u>Initiate ABCs (airway, breathing, circulation) while cooling efforts are initiated:</u>

- Move casualty from heat.

- Remove victim's clothing.

- Initial IV bolus of Ringer's Lactate or Normal Saline. Monitor for development of pulmonary edema.

- Avoid potassium supplementation until urine output is assured.

- Monitor temperature using rectal thermometer if available. Do not attempt to take an oral temperature in a confused or combative person.

- Seizures may occur, especially with cooling, and should be immediately controlled with IV benzodiazepine (lorazepam is preferred).

<u>Rapid cooling is mandatory:</u>

- Evaporative cooling is effective and easiest to perform using fans blowing cooler air and continuous tepid water spray. Elevating the patient on a mesh litter will improve airflow beneath the patient and enhance cooling. (Avoid cold water and cooling the skin below 30°C (86°F) as this can cause peripheral vasoconstriction and shivering.)

- Ice water immersion is effective and favored by some. It can, however, be difficult to manage an obtunded or pediatric casualty. It is better suited for adult victims suffering from exertional heat stroke. There is a slightly higher mortality rate when used for victims of classic heat stroke.

- Whole-body ice packing involves covering the trunk and extremities with crushed ice. The undesired effect of cutaneous vasoconstriction can be reduced by vigorous massage of the skin or alternating with evaporative methods.

- **Strategic ice packing involves placing ice packs in axillae, groin, and around the anterior neck.**

- Invasive methods include ice-water gastric and peritoneal lavage and should, if used, supplement the non-invasive methods. They require advanced technical expertise and can result in water intoxication.

- Do NOT use alcohol baths. Avoid antipyretics as these may cause more liver damage.

- Actively cool until core temperature equals 39°C (102°F). Continued cooling will cause hypothermia.

- After cooling, monitor temperature closely as patients can have difficulty with thermoregulation for a few days.

TREATMENT TIP:

The absence of CNS disturbances distinguishes heat exhaustion from heat stroke.

	Sweating	Core temp >38.3°C (101°F)	End-organ damage	CNS changes
Heat syncope	●			
Heat cramps	●	+/-		
Heat tetany	●	+/-		
Heat exhaustion	●	●		
Heat injury	●	●	●	
Heat stroke	+/-	●	●	●

Fluid Hydration for Rescuers

Enforcing fluid hydration in rescuers is a leadership responsibility.

- Leaders must supervise and verify water intake. Most rescuers tend not to drink enough and will not voluntarily stop work to drink.
- **Lack of thirst is NOT a reliable indication of hydration!**
- Monitor for the following, which may be symptoms of dehydration and impending heat injury:

    o Urine color (dilute vs. dark) and frequency of urination

    o Dizziness

    o Headache, nausea, vomiting

    o Confusion and euphoria

    o Abdominal pain

    o Muscle cramps

WORLD HEALTH ORGANIZATION REHYDRATION FORMULA:

- A Pinch of Salt
- A Handful of Sugar
- A Liter of Water

Common Foods and Their Approximate Salt Content

Food or Beverage Item	Serving Size	Sodium (mg)
Chicken Noodle Soup or Bouillon	1 cup (8oz.)/236 mL	1107
Dill Pickle	1 pickle (medium)	1008
Tomato Juice	1 cup	882
Salted Pretzels	1 oz. (28 g)	483
Corn Flakes Cereal	1 cup	281
Gatorade®	1 cup	110
Soda	1 cup	2–8
Water	1 cup	7

Summary

Heat-related illnesses are a significant cause of morbidity and mortality in many disasters and affect both responders and victims. Prevention and early recognition of heat-related conditions are the key to preventing life-threatening conditions such as heat stroke.

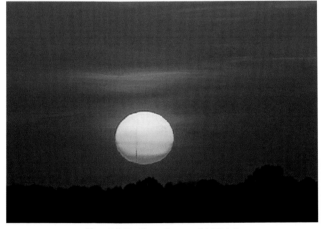

Fig. 22.3 Courtesy of NOAA

KEY POINTS

 Heat stroke is a medical emergency requiring aggressive medical interventions.

 Many medicines increase an individual's susceptibility to heat-related illnesses.

 Hydration, preferably oral, is the key to prevention of heat-related illnesses.

 Disaster victims and responders are both vulnerable to heat-related conditions.

Cold Injuries

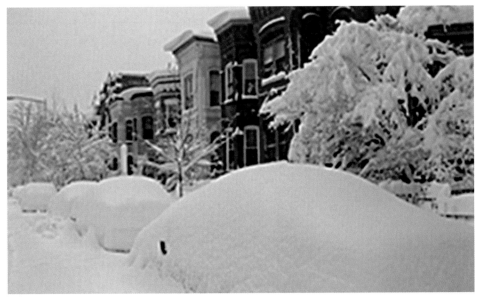

Fig. 23.1 Washington, DC Snowstorm, Courtesy of NOAA (2010)

CASE SCENARIO

Winter storms cause significant morbidity and mortality not only from cold injuries and hypothermia but from weather-related traumatic injuries. In February, 2010, an historic snowstorm in Washington, DC and the Mid-Atlantic States, dubbed "Snowmageddon," left the region paralyzed by a blizzard. Hundreds of thousands of individuals were left without power, and roads were impossible to navigate. EMS experienced a dramatic increase in 911 calls for cold-related conditions and injuries.

Introduction

Disaster casualties and providers alike are at risk for the spectrum of cold injuries, ranging from local tissue injuries such as frostnip, frostbite, and trench foot, to systemic injury caused by hypothermia. Local tissue injury due to cold may be freezing or non-freezing.

Pathophysiology

When the body begins to cool, a host of *physiological* defense mechanisms begin in order to conserve heat:

- Peripheral vasoconstriction
- Peripheral blood shunts to the body core (internal organs)
- Autonomic nervous system stimulation
- *Shivering* (involuntary muscle contractions) increases basal metabolism 3-5 fold and is extremely important in thermogenesis (limited to 2 hours and blunted/shortened by glycogen deprivation, alcohol/drugs, fatigue). Response is maximum at 35°C (95°F) and extinguished at 31°C (87.8°F). Without shivering, the individual's body temperature plummets.

Behavioral changes occur as well. Numbing cold depresses the central nervous system. With increasing hypothermia, an individual may experience:

- Confusion
- Impaired memory and judgment
- Slurred speech
- Decreased consciousness

The severity of cold injury is a function of:

- Absolute temperature
- Duration of exposure
- Wind velocity
- Environmental conditions (conductive heat loss increased 5-fold if clothing is wet, 25-fold in water)
- The individual's general health

Other predisposing factors include:

- Inadequate insulation from the cold and wind
- Altitude
- Age

TREATMENT ALERT!

Decreases in blood flow caused by shock or tight-fitting clothes may predispose to cold injury.

FIELD OBSERVATION

Poor judgement is a common cause of death from hypothermia.

- Fatigue or sleep deprivation

- Hypoxia

- Tobacco use

- Water immersion

- Shock

- Fractures, spinal cord injury

- Raynaud's Disease

- Cerebrovascular accident

- Diabetic ketoacidosis

- Hypoglycemia

- Hypothyroidism

- Uremia

- Associated trauma

- Dehydration

- Poor nutrition

- Peripheral vascular disease

- Alcohol and drugs

- Previous cold injury

- Warm climate residence

- Constriction (dressings/clothing/swelling)

- Cognitive impairment-mental illness, intoxication, dementia, cerebral edema, fear/panic

Accidental Hypothermia

Accidental hypothermia occurs in a variety of settings and in all seasons. Exposure to cold and exhaustion are common causes of hypothermia in disasters. Wetness and wind are a more lethal combination than dry cold alone.

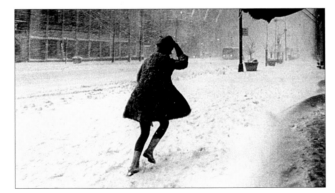

Fig. 23.2 Winter blizzard, Courtesy of NOAA

FIELD OBSERVATION

- Immersion hypothermia is characterized by rapid onset and faster rate of cooling.
- Heat loss is 25 times greater in water than in air.

RISK ALERT!

- Hypothermic casualties have increased cardiovascular instability.

- Slight patient movements or jarring—(e.g., CPR, intubation, and rough transport) may precipitate ventricular fibrillation.

- **Mild hypothermia** ranges between 32–35°C (89.6–95°F). Symptoms include:
    - o Shivering
    - o Loss of motor coordination
    - o Lethargy
    - o Confusion
    - o Tachycardia
    - o Amnesia/poor judgment
    - o Dysarthria/ataxia/clumsiness

- **Moderate hypothermia** ranges from 30–32°C (86–89.6°F). Symptoms include:
    - o Decreased shivering
    - o Loss of consciousness
    - o Hypotension
    - o Bradycardia
    - o Decreased respirations
    - o Atrial arrhythmias

- **Severe hypothermia** is below 30°C (86°F). Symptoms include:
    - o Coma with dilated pupils
    - o Hypotension
    - o Bradycardia
    - o Loss of muscle tone
    - o Life-threatening cardiac arrhythmias
    - o Depressed or absent respirations
    - o Decreased cardiac output

Cold Immersion

1. Cold Shock Response (1-2 minutes) - Water T <20°C (68°F)

    a. Immediate gasping response

    b. Inability to breath-hold

    c. Hyperventilation

    d. Increased cardiac output, heart rate, and blood pressure with increased cardiac workload

2. Cold Incapacitation (3-15 minutes)–Loss of fine and gross motor coordination and power for self-rescue

3. Hypothermia (>30 minutes)-loss of consciousness after 1 hour and asystole at 2 hours

4. Collapse at Rescue (20% death rate in live "recoveries")

    a. **Afterdrop-continued decline in core temperature after removal from cold up to 5-6°C (9-10°F)**

    b. Collapse of arterial pressure-loss of "hydrostatic squeeze"

    c. Ventricular fibrillation

RISK ALERT!

Without personal floatation devices, drowning is the most likely cause of death with cold water immersion.

Clinical Evaluation of Casualties

Special thermometers capable of registering low temperatures are necessary in the hypothermic patient. Standard thermometers are not accurate at low temperatures. Rectal temperatures and esophageal temperature probes more closely reflect the body's core temperature. Oral and axillary temperatures are unreliable.

Selected Characteristics of Mild, Moderate, and Severe Hypothermia

Stage	Core Temp °C		Core Temp °F	Effects
Mild	37.6		99.7	Normal rectal temperature
	34.0		93.2	Amnesia, difficulty speaking, and poor judgment; normal blood pressure; increased respiration; tachycardia
Moderate	31.0		87.8	**Extinguished shivering thermogenesis**
	30.0		86.0	Atrial fibrillation and other arrhythmias
	29.0		84.2	Progressive decrease in the level of consciousness, pulse, and respiration; pupils dilated
	27.0		80.6	Loss of reflexes and voluntary motion
Severe	26.0		78.8	No response to pain
	23.0		73.4	No corneal or oculocephalic reflexes; areflexia
	22.0		71.6	Maximum risk of ventricular fibrillation
	18.0		64.4	Asystole
	13.7		56.8	Lowest adult accidental hypothermia survival

TREATMENT TIP:

Plastic garbage bags can be used as a vapor barrier for hypothermia casualties.

Treatment

- **Prevent further heat loss and provide heat!**
- Insulate the casualty from the wind and cold ground.
- Remove all freezing and wet clothes.
- Put the casualty in a dry sleeping bag or wrap with dry blankets; cover with a vapor barrier.
- Cover the head with a wool cap or other warm item.
- Keep patient horizontal (avoid orthostatic hypotension, especially if immersion injury)
- **Never leave a hypothermia casualty alone.**

Treatment methods of rewarming are based upon the severity of hypothermia. These include:

- Passive external rewarming
- Active external rewarming
- Active core or internal rewarming

Passive external rewarming is sufficient for most cases of <u>mild</u> hypothermia, and rewarms the victim by utilizing:

- Blankets
- Other dry insulating material (from ground up)
- Oxygen if at altitude
- Warm carbohydrate fluids orally if mental status intact
- A warm environment with wind and vapor barriers
- Exercise if feasible

Active external rewarming delivers heat externally to the skin and increases body temperature slowly. Methods include:

- Heating blankets
- Hot water bottles on axillae, groin and neck (protect skin with fleece to avoid burns)
- Heating lamps/radiant heat
- Hot circulating baths 40°C (104°F) (difficulties in simultaneous monitoring/resuscitation and risk of "core afterdrop" if unable to maintain peripheral vasoconstriction)
- Plumbed garments with circulated warm fluid
- Forced circulated hot air
- Arteriovenous anastomosis rewarming, possibly with negative pressure application (exogenous heat 44-45°C (111.2-113°F) applied to distal extremities below knees and elbows, opening arteriovenous anastomoses, promoting patient comfort, and decreasing "core afterdrop").

Active core rewarming includes invasive methods of rewarming that deliver heat to the core of the body. It can be accomplished in several ways:

- Airway rewarming with heated, humidified oxygen 40-45°C, (104-113°F), Rewarming rate 1.5-2°C/hr (2.7-3.6°F/hr)
- Heated infusions of intravenous fluids 40-42°C (104-107.6°F), 500 mL D5NS

> **TREATMENT TIP:**
>
> In the field, active external rewarming may be accomplished by the use of another individual's body heat (e.g., a warm rescuer and a cold victim placed together in a sleeping bag).

> **RISK ALERT!**
>
> Active core rewarming is necessary in the presence of cardiovascular instability, severe hypothermia, and casualties who fail to warm with other methods.

> **TREATMENT TIP:**
>
> Heated, humidified oxygen inhalation is an excellent method for airway rewarming. Rewarming rates are greater when oxygen is administered via endotracheal tube than by mask.

- Heated irrigations:
    - o Gastric lavage (patient should be intubated)
    - o Mediastinal irrigation
    - o Thoracic lavage
    - o Peritoneal lavage
    - o Bladder/colonic irrigation
- Hemodialysis
- Extracorporeal blood warming

Treatment for Severe Hypothermia

If a monitor or automated external defibrillator indicates ventricular fibrillation or pulseless ventricular tachycardia, deliver 1 set of 3 stacked shocks. **Defibrillation is rarely effective if core T <30°C (86°F).** If the core temperature cannot be determined or is above 30°C (86°F), treat the patient as if normothermic.

Ventricular fibrillation is exceedingly difficult to treat in the severely hypothermic patient and is often refractory to conventional treatment.

CPR has no significant effect on outcome in many severely hypothermic casualties. Do not perform CPR if the patient is breathing or has a pulse. Suggested guidelines from the literature for not initiating CPR are:

- Cold-water submersion for patients underwater for more than 1 hour
- Hypothermic patient with core temperature of <15.5°C (59.9°F)
- Frozen patients (e.g., ice in the airway)
- Victim with stiff chest wall-making compressions impossible
- Rescuer exhaustion or danger
- Associated lethal injuries
- Signs of death:
    - o Airway and chest frozen
    - o Core temperature less than 15.5°C (59.9°F) or same as environment
    - o Potassium >10
    - o Elevated ammonia level
    - o Flat EEG with T>22°C (71.6°F)

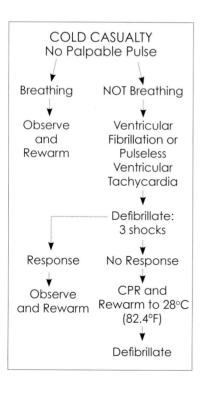

COLD CASUALTY
No Palpable Pulse

Breathing → Observe and Rewarm

NOT Breathing → Ventricular Fibrillation or Pulseless Ventricular Tachycardia → Defibrillate: 3 shocks

Response → Observe and Rewarm

No Response → CPR and Rewarm to 28°C (82.4°F) → Defibrillate

Local Cold Injuries

Non-Freezing Injuries

Local non-freezing injuries include chilblains (pernio), and trench (Immersion) foot/hand.

Chilblains (or Pernio)

Chilblains is primarily a dermatological manifestation of chronic exposure to damp or dry cold.

- **Setting:** bare skin in cold, windy weather environments
- **Location:** face, anterior tibial surface, dorsum of hands or feet, and other chronically exposed areas not protected from the cold
- **Signs:** pruritic, red-purple skin lesions (papules, macules, plaques, or nodules)

Trench (or Immersion) Foot/Hand

This non-freezing injury of the extremities occurs from chronic exposure to cold above freezing temperatures 1.6°–10°C (35-50°F) and wet conditions. Vasoconstriction of arterioles results in loss of heat and oxygen supply to surface tissues.

- **Setting:** immobility in cold, wet, windy weather environments
- **Signs:** initial numbness and cold progress to hyperemia in 24-28 hours; painful burning, edema, blistering, redness, ecchymosis, and ulcerations. Skin initially can appear cold, waxy, mottled, sodden, and friable with dark burgundy/blue splotches. Later, it can be red, hot, and blistered.
- **Prevention:** Avoid tight footwear, change socks at least once a day, and air dry and massage feet every 4 hours.
- **Treatment:** Dry and warm feet, oral hydration, ibuprofen every 6 hours, evacuation of victim.

Freezing Injuries

Local freezing injuries include frostnip and frostbite.

Frostnip

Frostnip is a superficial injury involving the skin surface and is the mildest form of cold injury. It causes numbness with a bluish-white discoloration of the affected body parts. Frostnip generally does not have sequela, although chronic frostnip exposure may lead to fat pad loss or atrophy. Treatment is simply rewarming.

Frostbite

Frostbite refers to a local freezing injury from intracellular ice crystal formations and microvascular occlusion, resulting in tissue anoxia. Frostbite is an ischemic injury and may be *superficial* or *deep*. It is often difficult to differentiate between superficial and deep injuries.

Superficial frostbite involves the skin, but not underlying fat and tissues. It is non-blanching to light-pressure, appears waxy, and is still soft and pliable. The subject complains of an aching or burning pain with tingling, numbness, and impaired movement.

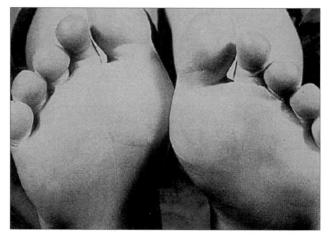

Fig. 23.3 Frostbite with edema and cyanosis,
Courtesy of Department of Defense

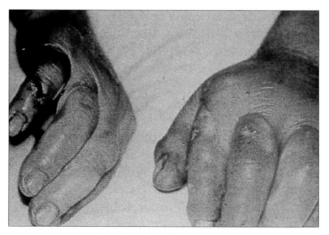

Fig. 23.4 Frostbite blebs,
Courtesy of Department of Defense

Deep frostbite involves the skin, connective tissue, muscles, tendons, nerves, and bones. Initially, the affected body part is hard, cold, white, and anesthetic. The tissue becomes cyanotic and ecchymotic during thawing. The extremity feels like a "block of wood" and cannot be depressed. Signs of deep frostbite include purple-colored "wooden skin" with non-blanching cyanosis and small blisters filled with hemorrhagic fluid.

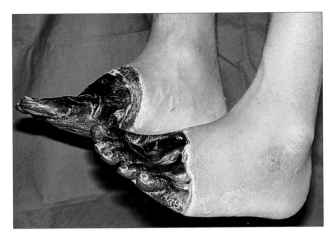

Fig. 23.5 Deep Frostbite

Treatment of Frostbite Injuries

- **Rapid rewarming is essential!** An immersion bath at 40°C (104°F) is the preferred method of rewarming, if available. Refreezing after partial warming may lead to neurological complications in the affected areas.

Important treatment protocols include:

- Do not break blisters.
- Do not rub or massage tissue or apply wet creams or dressings.
- Provide tetanus prophylaxis.
- Protect and cradle the extremity post-thawing by elevating the extremity.
- Place cotton padding between the toes and fingers.
- Administer non-steroidal anti-inflammatory agents such as ibuprofen 400 mg orally every 6 hours or ketorolac (Toradol®) 30 mg every 8-12 hours IV. These medicines will relieve pain and may decrease the extent of injury.
- Do not apply tight bandages.
- Do not debride frostbite.

RISK ALERT!

Avoid the freeze-thaw-refreeze cycle. Wait until the casualty is in a warm environment before thawing the extremities.

Prevention of Local Cold Injuries

Since there is not a good cure for cold injuries, prevention is critical. Command guidance, proper shelter, clothing, and nutrition are essential. Other preventative measures include:

- Wearing clothes loosely and in layers. Air space between clothes conserves heat. Avoid tight boots/too many socks.
- Use undergarments that "wick" away the moisture from the body.
- Choose outerwear that "breathes," allowing moisture to escape and resisting moisture from entering.
- Preserve body heat by covering head, neck, and face.
- Mittens are better than gloves. Lightweight thin gloves can be worn under mittens for short occasions when increased dexterity is needed in extreme cold environments.
- Keep clothing dry and clean. Store clothing dry in 1 - 2 gallon plastic bags.
- Stay well-hydrated.
- Maintain metabolic heat production with adequate caloric intake.
- Maintain "Hunting Response" or cold-induced vasodilatation by avoiding dehydration and alcohol and using supplemental oxygen when potentially hypoxic at extreme altitude.
- Do not become overtired in the cold. Avoid overexertion and sweating.
- Do not work in wet clothes.
- Use a buddy system to watch for signs of cold injury.

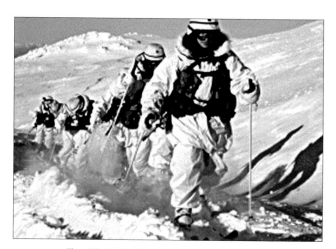

Fig. 23.6 Cold weather deployment,
Courtesy of Department of Defense

Preparing Hypothermic Casualties for Transport

- Remove wet clothing from casualty.

- Stabilize injuries (e.g., spine), and cover open wounds.

- Start IV infusion, if possible.

- Initiate active external warming.

- Wrap casualty with available insulating materials (blankets, etc.)

- Protect patient and staff from cold rotor-wash.

Summary

Weather-related disasters such as severe blizzards present a significant risk for cold injuries, ranging from local tissue injuries to severe hypothermia. Prompt recognition and treatment of the spectrum of cold injuries will decrease morbidity and mortality in both victims and disaster responders.

KEY POINTS

 Casualties with hypothermia often die from poor judgment rather than from the effects of the hypothermia.

 Ventricular fibrillation is difficult to treat in the hypothermic patient and resistant to many standard therapeutic modalities.

 Avoid the freeze-thaw-refreeze cycle. Refreezing after partial warming may lead to significant neurological deficits in the affected extremity.

Environmental Toxicology

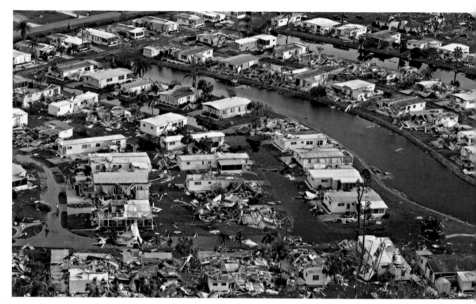

Fig. 24.1 Hurricane Katrina (2005)

CASE SCENARIO

A 37-year-old man, member of a disaster team responding to a devastating hurricane, was admitted to a field hospital with difficulty breathing, airway compromise, and hypotension. He was awake, alert, oriented, and extremely agitated. Prior to arrival, he received 1 mg of epinephrine subcutaneous (SC) and 50 mg of diphenhydramine intramuscularly (IM) in the field. On arrival, he had the following vital signs: blood pressure 90/45, pulse 130, respiratory rate 38, and temperature 98.8° F. Pulse oximetry was 95%.

Treatment was initiated for a presumptive diagnosis of an anaphylactic reaction from an insect bite. The patient received multiple 90 mcg inhalations of albuterol and 125 mg of intravenous (IV) methylprednisolone. A raised red lesion with a stinger at the center was found on the patient's right forearm. The stinger was removed, and the patient gradually improved to full recovery and normal vital signs after several hours.

Introduction

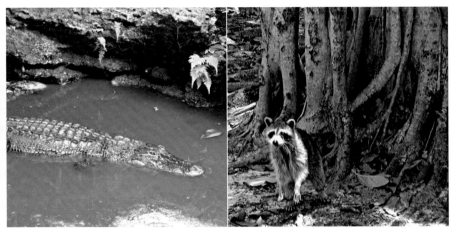

Figs. 24.2, 24.3 Environmental Challenges

Disasters can occur in any type of climate or environment. Be it desert, mountain, forest, or sea, every disaster scenario holds the potential for exposure to environmental toxins or poisons. The more austere the environment and the more infrastructure becomes disrupted, the greater the likelihood that rescuers will face toxicological emergencies. Exposures range from insect stings and bites to direct contact with plants or ingestion of toxic plants if there is a disruption of the food supply. These hazards can pose additional threats beyond the primary disaster scene, resulting in increased morbidity and mortality both to disaster victims and responders. Being able to prevent, identify, and treat a variety of poisonous flora and fauna are essential skills for any disaster responder.

Preparation for Disasters

Disaster responders should research geographic-specific exposures and be aware of such hazards. Key interventions to prevent envenomization (injection of a poisonous material by sting, spine, bite, or other similar means) include:

- Ensure appropriate medications to handle potential exposures are included in the pharmaceutical cache.
- Take steps to prevent envenomization and reduce exposure, including wearing appropriate clothing.
- Avoid ingestion of local plants, berries, and mushrooms.
- Know the right interventions for a given toxin in a timely fashion.

Insects

A. Spiders

1. Black Widow Spiders (Latrodectus)

Black (or brown) widow spiders are found in virtually every state in the United States (USA). They are black spiders with the more potent females often bearing a classic red hourglass on their ventral abdomen.

Clinical Characteristics

Bites are often unnoticed at the time of inoculation. Within minutes to hours, victims will experience cramping and pain of large muscle groups, most commonly in the back, thighs, and abdomen. **It has even been misdiagnosed as appendicitis!** The venom is a neurotoxin, and, if untreated, may take days to weeks to completely resolve.

Treatment

- Treatment is mostly supportive with opioids for pain and muscle relaxants or benzodiazepines.
- Calcium has been used in the past with mixed results and is rarely used anymore.
- Antivenom is reserved for cases refractory to opioid pain control or with worsening symptoms. One to two vials is often all that is required for complete reversal of symptoms. This treatment is not without its own risks. It is a horse serum-derived product and carries the risk of allergy and anaphylaxis.
- Tetanus status should be updated in black widow bite victims.

2. Brown Recluse Spiders (Loxosceles)

Brown recluse spiders are endemic to the southern United States. They are often mistakenly assumed to be present outside their normal distribution. Methicillin-resistant *Staphylococcus aureus* (MRSA) and other necrotic skin lesions can be incorrectly diagnosed as brown-recluse envenomization.

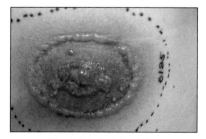

Fig. 24.4 Spider bite

Clinical Characteristics

Spiders bite in self-defense and are at first unnoticed. A pruritic papule develops, and toxic agents in the venom cause necrotic ulcers, which are often disfiguring and may become chronic. Wounds may have a 'bulls-eye' appearance around the central necrotic lesion. Common areas for bites are the wrist and ankle, where a spider may become caught in a sock or sleeve. Multiple lesions should raise suspicion of an infectious or self-inflicted (skin-popping) etiology. Systemic envenomization is rare but possible. Patients may develop hemolysis and become severely ill but most cases, however, have mild presentations.

Treatment

- Supportive treatment, including cold compresses to the site and wound care.
- Dapsone, while controversial, has been used in an attempt to block migration of white blood cells to the center of the necrotic zone.
- Antibiotics are unnecessary unless superinfection occurs.
- There is no role for steroid use, as most cases are self-limited.
- Tetanus status should be updated.

B. Hymenoptera: Bees, Wasps, Hornets

Among the order Hymenoptera ("membranous wings"), the honeybee is the only member that leaves a stinger with venom behind. These insects often attack in swarms, and victims are prone to multiple stings. The Africanized honeybee is virtually indistinguishable from its European counterpart. However, they display much more aggressive behavior. Victims of an Africanized colony may present with hundreds to thousands of stings.

Clinical Characteristics

After a sting, the onset of effect is almost immediate with burning and stinging at the local site. In most individuals, erythema and pain are the only complications. **Allergic individuals, up to 2% of the population, are prone to anaphylaxis from bee stings.**

Treatment

- If present, stingers should be removed as quickly as possible to reduce envenomization. This may be performed by scraping at the site with a piece of firm plastic such as a credit card.

- Cold compresses or ice packs applied to affected areas provide symptomatic relief.

Strict monitoring and stabilization of ABCs is mandatory to prevent shock in *anaphylactic reactions*. **People exhibiting signs and symptoms of anaphylactic shock should be treated with epinephrine, antihistamines and corticosteroids.**

C. Fire Ants

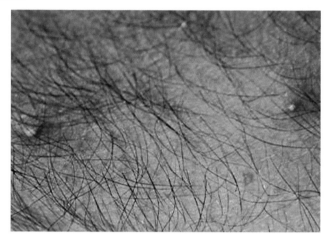

Fig. 24.5 Fire ant bites

Fire ants have a worldwide distribution with more than 250 species. Though fire ants may bite with their mandibles, the injection of alkaline venom occurs through a stinger on the caudal end of the abdomen. Bites have a characteristic circular pattern from repeated stinging while the ant rotates around the embedded mandible.

Clinical Characteristics
Most victims experience local pain and raised papules, which become slightly pustular over the next 12-48 hours. Scratched lesions are prone to local infection.

Treatment
- Supportive treatment with topical steroids or oral antihistamines.
- Antibiotics are necessary only when lesions become superinfected.

Some individuals are severely allergic to the venom of fire ants and may experience anaphylactic symptoms and merit appropriate treatment.

Snakes

A. Rattlesnakes (Crotalinae)

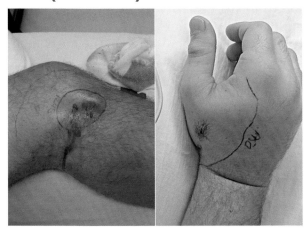

Figs. 24.6, 24.7 Rattlesnake Bites

Rattlesnakes (genus *Crotalus*), cottonmouth (*Sistrurus*, aka water moccasin), and copperhead (*Agkistrodon*) make up the subfamily crotalinae. The snakes are characterized by hinged fangs capable of injecting venom from venom sacs. Pits located between the nostril and eyes are used as a sensing device for tracking prey and give rise to the alternative name "pit viper".

Clinical Characteristics

Venom has multiple components designed to predigest prey. Rapidly advancing soft tissue swelling may occur. Progressive swelling and myonecrosis may result in compartment syndrome, loss of tissue, and long-term disability if not treated. Repeated measurements are necessary to determine the progression of symptoms and the need for ongoing therapy. Thrombocytopenia and coagulopathy may progress to a disseminated intravascular coagulopathy. Some venoms, notably that of the Mojave rattlesnake, may give rise to neurotoxic symptoms such as muscle fasciculations. Severe envenomization results in hypotension and requires immediate intervention.

Treatment

- Pretreatment with antibiotics, steroids, and antihistamines is usually unnecessary.

- **The current available antivenom (Crofab) is an ovine-derived Fab.** Initial treatment is 4-6 vials IV over an hour. If initial control is not obtained, an additional 4-6 vials may be given. Maintenance dosing of 2 vials every 6 hours for 3 additional doses (6 vials) is recommended, but may be skipped in mild cases where there is clearly no risk of progression of symptoms.

271

- Symptomatic and supportive care with particular attention to airway and circulation.

- **Expert consultation in the treatment of snakebites is highly recommended for all exposures.**

- Copperhead bites may often be observed without the need for antivenom administration.

- Update tetanus status.

B. Elapidae

Coral snakes are the only US elapid. These are brightly colored snakes with red, yellow, and black bands encircling the snake. Similar appearing species such as the king snake and scarlet king snake give rise to the adage: **"red on yellow, kill a fellow; red on black, venom lack"**. Another distinguishing factor of the US coral is their black nose. Exceptions to these general rules, however, do exist even within the United States. The snakes are generally docile and usually only bite when provoked. Coral snakes lack fangs and attach with a chewing motion. Patients have reported a Velcro-like sensation when pulling off a biting snake.

Clinical Characteristics
About a third of patients exhibit local swelling at the site of the bite. The venom is primarily a neurotoxin, and victims may exhibit localized numbness and tingling at the bite site. Nausea and vomiting are common. Paralysis of bulbar musculature results in inability to handle oral secretions and may result in aspiration pneumonia. Paralysis of the muscles of respiration may lead to respiratory failure.

Treatment
- Intubation for airway protection should be performed early in patients with a diminished gag reflex or inability to handle oral secretions.

- Antivenom is effective if administered prior to the onset of symptoms. Once symptoms have developed, antivenin becomes less effective as it does not appear to reverse symptoms once they occur. Symptoms may occur within the first hour or may be delayed for more than 8 hours. Initial dose of antivenom is 3 to 5 vials.

- Patients that do not get treatment with antivenom may require airway protection and ventilator assistance for up to 6 weeks.

- Prophylactic antibiotics and steroids are unnecessary.

- Tetanus status should be updated.

Marine Toxic Exposures

A. Jellyfish, Portuguese Man-of-War

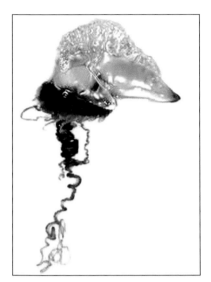

*Fig. 24.8 Portuguese Man-of-War,
Courtesy of NOAA*

Jellyfish are coelenterates, which can be found in all of the world's oceans. Humans may come in contact with tentacles, which contain specialized cells called nematocysts that inject venom. The Portuguese man-of-war (*Physalia*) is a colonial organism and technically not considered a jellyfish. However, envenomization from this organism is clinically indistinguishable from that of the jellyfish. The long tentacles of the Portuguese Man-of-War give rise to the characteristic lesions shown in the picture below.

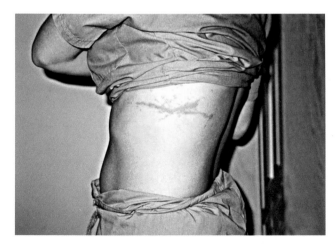

Fig. 24.9 Portuguese Man-of-War bite

273

Clinical Characteristics

Victims are exposed when in marine environments and make cutaneous contact. The abrasion-like wound is painful, but can be life-threatening in massive envenomization or acute anaphylaxis. The box jellyfish of Australia *(Chironex fleckeri)* is the notable exception with immediate life-threatening toxicity that may require antivenom administration.

Treatment

- Avoidance is the primary way to avoid exposure, especially with physical barriers such as long-sleeve shirts, skin suits, etc.

- Treatment consists of 3 phases: Inactivation of nematocysts, decontamination and removal of residual tentacle, and symptomatic and supportive care.

- Vinegar (acetic acid) is the most common agent used for inactivation of nematocysts. Seawater may also be utilized as it is almost always more accessible than acetic acid. Placing the envenomized skin back into the sea water may be the best option if time to vinegar application will be delayed.

- Evidence suggests that topical lidocaine may also be useful both for inactivation of nematocysts and treatment of pain.

- Other agents such as alcohol, sodium bicarbonate, urine and ammonia are less useful and may actually increase nematocysts firing.

- Some studies suggest an increase in nematocysts firing and venom injection from the application of acetic acid to nematocysts from the Portuguese man-of-war.

- Decontamination should be performed via scraping over the wound with a smooth edge such as a credit card.

- The toxin is heat-labile. Analgesia may be obtained by immersing the affected extremity in hot water, 40-42° C. Care should be taken to avoid scalding.

- A commercially available product made to replicate the mucus secreted by clown fish has shown promise in decreasing stings.

B. Stingrays

Stingrays are a diverse group of cartilaginous fish, most of which bear barbed stingers on their long tails. They are most often encountered in coastal waters by swimmers, surfers, and scuba divers.

Clinical Characteristics

A reflex mechanism caused by stepping on the stingray causes their whiplike tails to stab and inject venom. The venom is typically more painful than life-threatening. Rare cases of intra-cardiac injection of the venom have resulted in death.

Treatment

- The toxin is heat-labile and should be treated by immersing the extremity in hot water at least 104°F, but care should be taken to avoid scalding of the skin with hot-water immersion.

- The wound should be cleaned and dressed and cleared of any foreign material as pieces of the tail sheath may break off into the wound.

- Prophylactic antibiotics are typically not needed.

- Tetanus status should be updated.

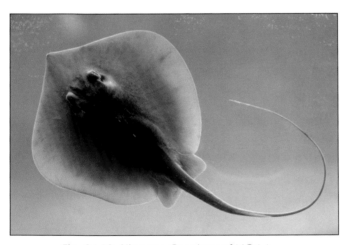

Fig. 24.10 Stingray, Courtesy of NOAA

C. Sea Urchins

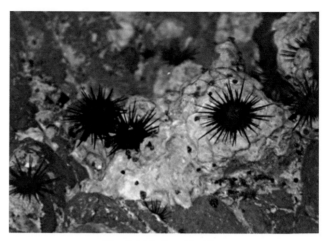

Fig. 24.11 Sea Urchins

Sea urchins are spine-covered animals commonly found in shallow waters in every ocean on the planet. If stepped-on or picked up, spines may embed in the skin and deliver a toxin to victims.

Clinical Characteristics
The spines are brittle and may break off into the wound. Calcifications and granulomatous reactions are common.

Treatment
- The removal of any visible spine within the wound may help avoid long-term complications.

- The heat-labile toxin of the sea urchin responds well to immersion in hot water.

D. Lionfish, Scorpionfish, Stonefish

Lionfish, scorpionfish, and stonefish contain erectile spines capable of injecting venom.

Clinical Characteristics
The envenomization is typically more painful than life-threatening, though, rarely can be more severe.

Treatment
- The toxin is heat-labile and pain is often responsive to the immersion in hot water, but care should be taken to avoid scalding.

Marine Toxic Ingestions

A. Ciguatera

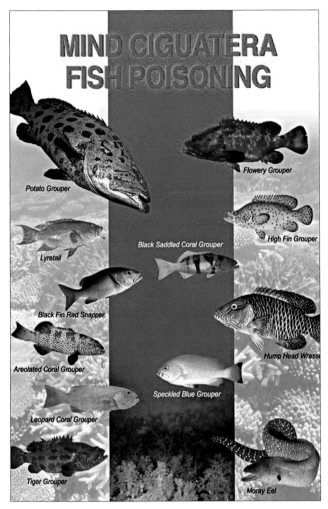

Fig. 24.12 Courtesy of Government of Hong Kong

Ciguatera is caused by the ingestion of preformed ciguatoxin in large carnivorous fish. The toxin is produced by a dynoflagellate, *Gamberdiscus toxicus*, which lives in the algae on coral reefs between the latitudes of 32 North and 32 South. Herbivorous fish feed off the algae, and are in turn consumed by carnivorous fish in which the toxin accumulates and is biotransformed. **Barracudas, snapper, parrotfish, grouper, triggerfish, and amberjack are among the most common fish.**

Clinical Characteristics

Symptoms may include a gastrointestinal phase with nausea, vomiting, and diarrhea and may include a brief quiescent phase prior to the onset of neurologic symptoms. Bizarre neurologic symptoms may include bradycardia, sensation of loose teeth, metallic taste, paresthesias, and the pathognomonic finding of hot-cold reversal. Intestinal phase may last a few hours up to two days. The neurologic symptoms typically last a few days with spontaneous resolution. Neuropsychiatric symptoms may last from weeks to years in a minority of patients with headaches, difficulty concentrating, asthenia, and malaise. Recurrences are common with the ingestion of alcohol, caffeine, and fatty foods such as peanuts. Though the disease is not considered contagious, sexual transmission via semen has resulted in pelvic pain in one patient.

Treatment

- Treatment, though controversial, is based on the administration of 2g/kg of mannitol, which appears to reduce the edema of affected neurons, and supportive care.

B. Scombroid

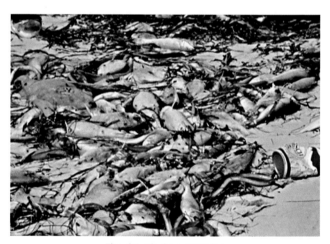

Fig. 24.13 Sea Urchins

Scombroid toxicity occurs after the ingestion of preformed histamine in improperly preserved fish. Bacteria in the flesh of the fish converts histidine to histamine.

Clinical Characteristics

Patients present with symptoms identical to an allergic reaction, and they are often difficult to distinguish. Flushing, swelling of the lips and tongue, and wheezing are common.

Treatment

- Because the histamine reaction is not related to allergy, there is a limited role for antihistamines or steroids.

- Epinephrine and beta-agonists are useful for treatment of wheezing.

Poisonous Plants

A. Plant Exposures: Poison Ivy, Oak, Sumac

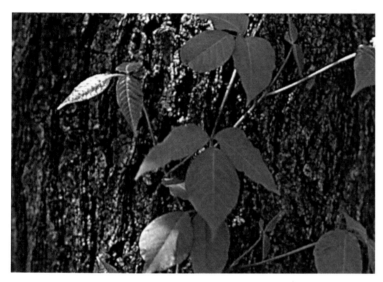

Fig. 24.14

The toxicodendron species cause Type 4 hypersensitivity reactions by direct contact with sap. The sap contains a toxin called Urushiol (also found in mangos) that is responsible for the contact dermatitis seen after exposure to these common plants. Exposure may not be limited to outdoor settings, as the toxin may be retained on clothing and equipment for weeks.

Clinical Characteristics

Patients with exposure to toxicodendrons present with an erythematous, blistering, and pruritic rash. The rash is made of macules, papules, and vesicles and often contains streaking where the patient has scratched. The rash appears on exposed skin to which the plant has come in contact.

Treatment

- Treatment involves symptomatic care with cool compresses, aveno baths, calamine lotion, caladryl lotion, topical corticosteroids, antihistamines, and, for severe cases, systemic corticosteroids. Patients that require oral steroids may need a course of 2-3 weeks with a taper. Commercial dose packs may not provide sufficient duration of therapy.

- Care should be taken to avoid the concurrent use of both topical and oral antihistamines as toxicity has been seen.

B. Toxic Plant Ingestions

1. Dieffenbachia, Philodendron, Elephant Ear

These calcium oxalate, crystal-containing plants with their broad leaves are ideal as houseplants, and may become toxic if ingested. These are most common small ingestions in curious children.

Clinical Characteristics

Patients report a crunching sensation when biting into a leaf. Calcium oxalate crystals embed in the oral mucosa and cause local irritation. Patients often present with swelling and erythema of the lips and oral mucosa. Drooling, difficulty swallowing, and difficult speech give rise to the nickname "dumbcane" for dieffenbachia.

Treatment

- Most cases are mild, but severe cases may result in airway obstruction and may necessitate an advanced airway.

2. Oleander, foxglove

Oleander and foxglove contain cardiac glycosides resembling digoxin. Most ingestions occur in children with less than a leaf and rarely result in clinical toxicity.

Clinical Charcteristics

The clinical syndrome and treatment mirrors that of digoxin toxicity. Nausea and vomiting are often the first sign of toxicity. Visual disturbances such as photophobia and color abnormalities are common. Increased cardiac contractility is the basis for the therapeutic use of digoxin in heart failure. Atrioventricular (AV) nodal block and increased vagal tone results in bradycardia with an increased PR interval on electrocardiogram (EKG). Virtually any electrocardiographic abnormality or dysrhythmia may be seen. Blockade of the Na-K ATPase pump results in hyperkalemia in the acute setting.

Treatment

- The treatment of toxicity is supportive care.

- Digoxin specific Fab (Digibind, Digifab) may be given for potassium levels greater than 5.0, hemodynamic instability (hypotension), or EKG findings of an unstable digoxin toxicity cardiac rhythm.

3. Rosary Pea, Castor Bean

The seed of the rosary pea (*Abrus precatorus*) and castor bean (*Ricinus communis*), often used as an ornament in necklaces or bracelets, contains a hard seed coat that protects against toxicity when swallowed whole. Both seeds contain toxalbumin, which enters the ribosome to prevent protein synthesis. Castor bean is the source of castor oil.

Clinical Charcteristics

When the seed coat has been breached, as in mastication, the clinical features are severe hemorrhagic gastroenteritis, which may lead to hypotension and shock. **Parenterally, toxalbumins are amoung the most potent toxins known.** Parenteral injection has been reported to cause a sepsis-like picture with high fever and shock. Castor bean has been weaponized for bioterrorism use by grounding to a very fine powder, which, when inhaled, can cause local necrosis and sloughing of the respiratory tract.

Treatment

- Treatment is symptomatic and supportive with attention to volume replacement.

4. Angel Trumpet, Jimson Weed

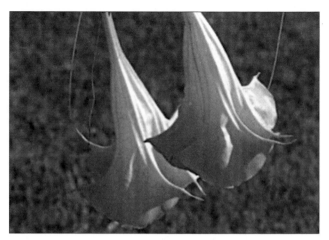

Fig.24.15 Angel Trumpet Flower

Jimsonweed (*Datura* species) grows as a low-lying bush with upturned bell-shaped flowers and seedpods. Angel trumpet (*Brugmansia* species) is more common in the southeastern United States and is often grown for ornamental purposes. It produces bell-like, 6-pointed, pendulous flowers. All parts of the plant contain anticholinergic alkaloids (atropine, scopolamine, and hyoscyamine).

Clinical Characteristics
Ingestion or smoking the plant results in clinical anticholinergic toxicity: tachycardia, flushing, mydriasis, urinary retention, drug mucosa, diminished bowel sounds, and hallucinations. **The adage "red as a beet, blind as a bat, hot as a hare, dry as a bone, and mad as a hatter" has been used to describe typical anticholinergic features.** With good symptomatic and supportive care mortality is rare.

Treatment
- The anticholinergic syndrome can be reversed with physostigmine. Its use is largely reserved for diagnostic purposes by many practitioners.

- The duration of toxicity from anticholinergic plant toxins is much longer than the duration of physostigmine.

- Benzodiazepines are useful for moderating tachycardia and behavioral management.

- Hyperthermia should be aggressively managed with physical means. There is no role for antipyretics such as aspirin or acetaminophen.

- Activated charcoal may be given early when gastrointestinal plant material such as seeds is suspected. Whole bowel irrigation (polyethylene glycol solution) may be used for decontamination provided the patient has not developed an ileus.

- Overflow incontinence is common. A Foley catheter is usually necessary for the treatment of urinary retention.

Summary

Toxic plant and animal species frequently add unexpected threats to disaster victims and responders alike. The clinical sequelae from these agents range from mild skin irritation to shock and even death. Preparations for specific environmental threats and swift interventions are key priorities for disaster responders. However, minimizing exposure is the most important tool when planning to handle environmental poisons.

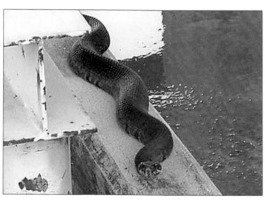 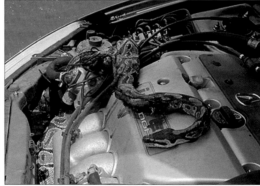

Figs. 24.16, 24.17 Unwelcome visitors to disaster site, Hurricane Katrina (2005)

KEY POINTS

 The more austere the environment, the more likely it is that toxicological emergencies will occur, both in disaster responders and victims.

 Medical personnel must possess knowledge of which toxins and poisons are treatable with antivenom and the time constraints related to administration of the antivenom.

 Pre-deployment knowledge of geographic-specific environmental hazards, if possible, is important in decreasing morbidity and mortality from environmental toxins/poisons.

Psychological Response to Disasters

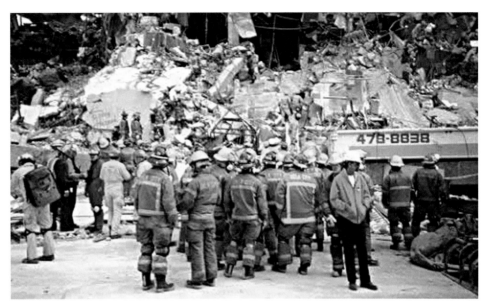

Fig. 25.1 Oklahoma City Bombing (1995), Courtesy of FEMA

CASE SCENARIO

The Oklahoma City bombing was a terrorist attack on the Alfred P. Murrah Federal Building in downtown Oklahoma City on April 10, 1995. A Ryder truck containing 4800 pounds of ammonium nitrate was detonated in front of the Murrah Federal Building which also housed a day care center. 168 individuals died, including 19 children under the age of 6 years. Over 680 people were injured. The region around the federal building also suffered significant damage. The terrorist was a war veteran and militia-movement sympathizer who intensely disliked the federal government. The psychological impact of this terrorist event was increased by the number of children killed, the presence of an American terrorist, and the location of the event in the heartland of the USA.

FORCES OF HARM

How individuals and communities respond and recover from disasters is a function of their interaction with specific "forces of harm", such as:

- Exposure to the hazard

- Extent and nature of the losses incurred

- Extent to which their lives are changed

Introduction

Psychological trauma and other adverse psychological sequelae are frequent components of events such as natural disasters, complex humanitarian disasters (e.g., refugee emergencies), and unintentional human-caused disasters. With terrorism, the objective is to inflict psychological pain, trauma, and disequilibrium.

It is important that planners, providers, and policy makers understand the importance of psychosocial issues. These are important, not only in the care of disaster victims and protection of disaster workers, but also in all aspects of the medical and public health response. These issues are also central in assuring that responders do not become victims themselves. Planners and providers will be more effective if they consider their own beliefs, biases, vulnerabilities, and fears.

Effective preparedness, response, and recovery depend on the successful integration of several systems within communities. Behavioral health service systems, medical care systems, public health systems, and emergency response systems are central. Sound preparedness, response, and recovery cannot take place in isolation.

Forces of Harm

How individuals and communities respond and recover from disasters is a function of their interaction with the events' forces of harm, specifically, their exposure to the hazard, the extent and nature of the losses incurred, and the extent to which their lives are changed (Norris, 2005; Shultz, et al, 2007). Examples include:

Exposure to Hazards

- ***Little or No Warning***
  Many disasters occur without warning. Warning allows individuals to take psychological and physical protective actions and provides a perception of control over the destructive event. A lack of warning deprives people of this opportunity and reduces perceived control, increasing the sense of helplessness, vulnerability, and disequilibrium.

- ***Physical and Psychological Proximity to the Event***
  Those physically and psychologically closer to the event (e.g., knowing someone in the impacted area or other associations with the disaster area or event) are at greater psychological risk.

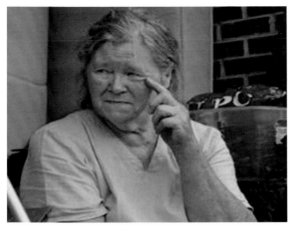

Fig.25.2 Hurricane Katrina (2005)

- **Diminished Health Status**

  Individuals who suffer from reduced health status are at increased psychological risk. Those who survive a terrorist event with injuries are often faced with long-term medical care, prolonged pain, physical rehabilitation, and multiple surgical interventions. Many of these individuals are at risk of becoming psychological casualties. Those whose health status was diminished prior to the event are also of concern.

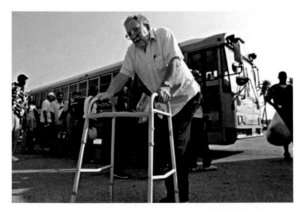

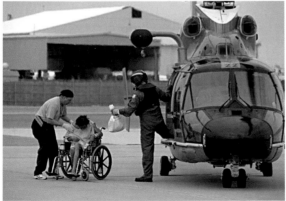

Figs.25.3, 25.4 Hurricane Katrina victims (2005)

PSYCHOLOGICAL RESPONSE

While most victims of a disaster will have some psychological reaction to it, most will **not** develop a diagnosable behavioral health disorder.

- ### *Serious Threat to Personal Safety*
  Events that expose individuals to personal health risks are associated with adverse psychological consequences.

- ### *Potential Unknown Health Effects*
  The fear of long-term health effects and the potential health effects on future generations increase psychological risk. This may come in the form of exposure to unknown noxious agents or agents with known adverse health effects. Terrorism involving biological, chemical or radioactive agents increases this risk factor.

- ### *Witnessing*
  Witnessing and/or prolonged exposure to destruction, gruesome scenes, mass casualties, and death have an increased risk of psychological harm. Those who are involved in the disaster response, rescue efforts, body recovery, and identification of remains are at particular risk.

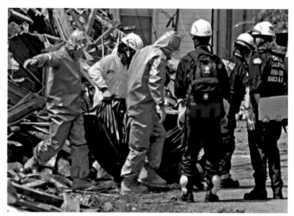

Fig.25.5 Search and rescue teams, Oklahoma City Bombing (1995), Courtesy of FEMA

Loss

Loss issues can impact psychological functioning and long-term outcome. The following types of loss increase psychological risk:

- Bereavement
- Separation from loved ones
- Loss of home and/or workplace
- Loss of possessions
- Loss of social support
- Loss of perceived control

Change

Types and magnitude of change can impact psychological functioning and long-term outcome. The following change factors can increase psychological risk:

- Physical displacement

- Change of school or employment

- Change of available community services

- Shortages, rationing, exploitation

- Financial hardship

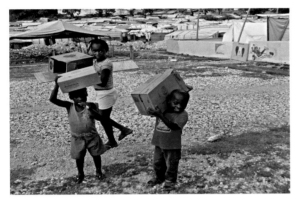

Fig.25.6 Displaced refugees, Haiti earthquake (2010)

Factors Impacting Psychological Response

Everyone who experiences a disaster, whether as a victim or as a responder, is affected by it. Fortunately, this does not mean that most will develop a mental health disorder, but it does mean that some type of psychological, physical, cognitive, and/or emotional response to the event(s) will occur in most exposed individuals. **Most, in fact, will not develop diagnosable behavioral health disorders.** Typically, symptoms decline over time.

Post-traumatic stress has sometimes been called the *common cold of psychiatry*. At some time in our lives, most people have experienced uncomfortable post-traumatic symptoms. In most cases, these decline and go away over time. For some, however, this is not the case and professional diagnosis and treatment are indicated.

Similarly, there are both individual and collective reactions that interact as individuals and communities recover from these extraordinary events.

TREATMENT TIP

Be conservative with diagnosing a stress or psychiatric diagnosis, especially in the early days and hours. This is especially important when the provider has limited contact with and history for the patient.

Those involved in both individual and community recovery should also be reminded that the rate and trajectory of recovery are highly variable, non-linear, and often do not occur in a synchronized or parallel manner. Factors impacting collective responses to disasters include:

- Degree of Community Disruption (physical and/or social)
  Some disasters occur leaving the social infrastructure intact. Others tear apart the very social fabric of communities, increasing adverse psychosocial consequences.

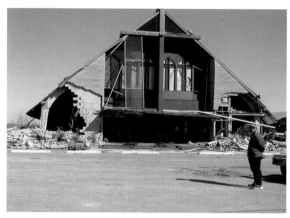

Fig.25.7 Church destroyed by Hurricane Katrina, (2005)

- Pre-disaster Family and Community Stability
  Those families and communities that functioned well prior to a disaster tend to fare better following the event.

- Community Leadership
  Communities in which leaders play a positive, decisive, and socially sensitive role in the hours and days following an event typically do better than those in which a leadership vacuum occurs or when leadership fails.

- Sensitivity of Recovery Efforts
  Recovery from a major disaster may require new housing, work, school, and other types of reconstruction. If recovery is delayed or insensitive, anger, disillusionment, and other negative psychological sequelae may occur. Recovery efforts that are sensitive to the cultural, socioeconomic, racial, and ethnic factors of the affected community usually result in a healthier recovery.

Epidemiological Research on Psychological Response to Disasters

Disaster research is difficult to conduct, and results are frequently inconclusive. Several studies, however, have identified a number of status factors that increase adverse psychological responses to disasters. These include:

- Gender: Women are at greater risk of post-traumatic stress disorder (PTSD) and major depression. Men are at greater risk of substance abuse.

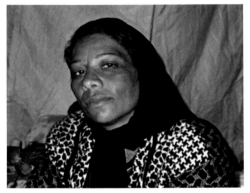

Fig.25.8 Iran earthquake (2005)

- Minority groups; individuals of low economic status.

- Family characteristics: Being an adult with children, being a female with a spouse, being a child of a dysfunctional parent, family instability.

- Psychiatric history: Prior psychiatric diagnosis, prior trauma, diminished cognitive ability, proneness to experience depression and anxiety.

- Adaptive skills and social support: Limited coping techniques, low belief in one's own ability to positively influence his/her future and limited social resources.

- Pre-disaster Functioning: Those who were functioning at a higher level before a disaster tend to fare better than those who were not.

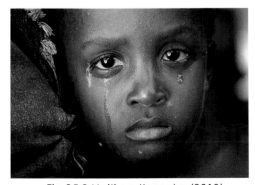

Fig.25.9 Haiti earthquake (2010)

291

TREATMENT TIP

Adverse psychological responses to disasters can include overlapping sub-clinical distress, diagnosable disorders, and increased health-risk behaviors.

Psychological Sequelae of Disasters

It is difficult to make generalizations about psychological sequelae following a disaster. While many people may exhibit signs of psychological stress, relatively few (typically 15%–25%) of those most directly impacted will subsequently develop a diagnosable mental disorder. Post-disaster responses are wide-ranging, from mild stress responses to full-blown PTSD, major depression, or acute stress disorders.

- ### Disaster-Related Stress

    Many disaster responders or victims will experience some constellation of physical, emotional, behavioral, and cognitive signs of stress during and following the disaster. Often, this stress can be significantly reduced and managed through education, provision of anticipatory guidance (what to expect next), and relatively informal counseling.

    Most individuals who have worked with disaster victims over time are struck by their resilience and ability to grow stronger by learning from the experience, developing new or improved coping skills, and establishing new or strengthened family and social supports.

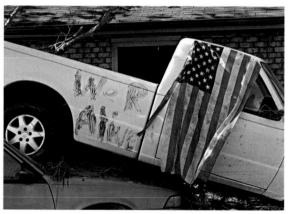

Fig.25.10 Hurricane Katrina (2005)

- **Mental Disorders**
  Typically, these include depression, acute stress disorders, PTSD, and phobias. Caution is encouraged regarding the temptation to look only for PTSD. In so doing, providers may miss other types of disorders.

  A special note regarding those people with pre-existing mental disorders. In many cases, these individuals do quite well in the early stages of response and recovery. They tend to have special problems as time goes on if the health, social, and vocational supports they required are not fully or rapidly restored. Providers should take care not to further stigmatize this population by diagnosing normal and expected stress as an exacerbation of their psychiatric illness.

- **Increased Health-Risk Behavior**
  These may include changes in smoking, substance use/abuse, risk taking (e.g., speeding and other dangerous behaviors).

Interventions

- Early interventions that include the following five characteristics appear to be most effective (Hobfol et al., 2007): **Promotion of a sense of safety, promotion of calming, promotion of a sense of self and collective efficacy, promotion of connectedness, and instilling hope.**

- Various forms of Psychological First Aid (PFA) are emerging as a promising early intervention. Goals of most models of PFA include engagement, safety and orientation, stabilization and self-regulation, and connectedness. It should be noted that while PFA is rapidly increasing in popularity, little research has been conducted regarding the efficacy of various models.

- Critical-incident stress management (CISM), which typically includes single-session critical incident stress debriefing (CISD) as one of its components, has been a very popular group intervention, especially among first responders. While most report feeling better following this type of experience, research on its efficacy (including potential harm) is mixed. The popularity of CISD-type interventions has declined as increasing evidence has emerged questioning its efficacy and even its potential to do harm. Other interventions, such as Eye Movement Desensitization and Reprocessing (EMDR) continue to be quite controversial.

- In cases where there is no diagnosed mental disorder, most agree that provision of educational materials that help people understand what they and their families are experiencing, and will experience in the future, is valuable. Information delivered in a manner that is clear, credible, and usable is an important intervention.

- Government programs to deal with large-scale psychological consequences typically focus upon education, brief crisis counseling, training of disaster-aid workers (e.g., clergy, teachers, disaster recovery workers, etc.), and referral when treatment is indicated.

- In cases where a mental disorder is diagnosed, psychotherapeutic interventions, such as cognitive behavioral therapy, have been found helpful as well as psychopharmacological interventions.

Worker Stress and Resilience

Disaster workers who choose to be involved in this type of work may gain great reward and satisfaction but can also become secondary victims of other adverse psychological sequelae. This can adversely affect their functioning during and after an event, including family and work relationships. Effectively managing stress and enhancing resilience requires effort on the part of workers as well as the organizations in which they work. Efforts to promote resilience and reduce occupational stress will be optimized when both groups take worker health seriously.

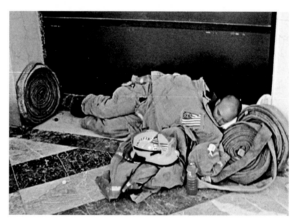

Fig.25.11 Search and rescue worker, Hurricane Katrina (2005)

Signs of Stress in Workers

Everyone experiences stress a bit differently. Some common signs of stress in workers include the following:

- **Physiological signs** of stress such as:

    o Fatigue, even after rest

    o Nausea

    o Fine motor tremors or tics

    o Paresthesias

    o Dizziness

    o Gastrointestinal (GI) upset

    o Heart palpitations

    o Choking or smothering sensations

- **Emotional signs** of stress such as:

    o Anxiety or feeling overwhelmed

    o Irritability

    o Unrealistic anticipation of harm to self or others

- **Cognitive signs** of stress such as:

    o Memory loss

    o Decision-making difficulties

    o Anomia (the inability to name common objects
    or familiar people)

    o Concentration problems or distractibility

    o Calculation difficulties

- **Behavioral signs** of stress such as:

    o Insomnia

    o Hypervigilance

    o Crying easily

    o Inappropriate humor

    o Ritualistic behavior (repetitive non-productive behavior)

ASSESSMENT TIP

Look for duration, intensity, multiplicity, and disruptive nature of stress signs. Very transient and minimally disruptive stress signs mean little in differentiating those who may need significant interventions.

Factors Contributing to Worker Stress

Many factors inherent in disaster situations contribute to worker stress. These include:

- Long work hours
- New professional challenges and working in an unfamiliar context
- Time pressures
- Multiple and/or conflicting priorities
- Exposure to traumatic experiences
- Unclear duration of event or deployment
- Fear of death, injury, or illness
- Role conflicts
- Balancing practice with bureaucracy and politics
- Reactions/responses of those who are being helped

Factors Mitigating Worker Stress

- Value and meaning of work, as well as public acknowledgment of its value
- Novelty of work
- Opportunity to be on the cutting edge
- The "rush" of the disaster environment

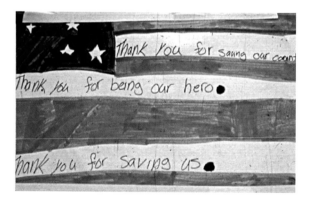

Fig.25.12 World Trade Center terrorist attack (2001)

Managing Worker Stress On-site

- Limit exposure to traumatic stimuli

- Reasonable hours

- Rest/sleep

- Reasonable diet

- Regular exercise program

- Private time

- Talking to somebody who understands

- Monitoring signs of stress

- An identifiable endpoint for involvement

Matrix of Responsibility

Both workers and the organizations in which they work are encouraged to collaborate on commitments in each of the cells of the following matrix (adapted from Shultz, Espinel, Flynn et al, 2007). Such pre-event planning and preparation will enhance the potential that efforts will be comprehensive, integrated, and appropriate to both job and organization.

Pre-event-Individual and Family (e.g., live a healthy lifestyle, learn stress management, promote family understanding of nature of disaster work)	**Pre-event-Organizational** (e.g., value worker health, plan for anticipated stress, implement policies that promote health)
Disaster Event-Individual and Family (e.g., self-monitoring, buddy-care, attempt healthy sleep and diet, communicate with family)	**Disaster Event-Organizational** (e.g., promote safe and supportive environment, monitor and confront stress in a way that does not stigmatize, allow relief/removal when warranted)
Post- Event-Individual and Family (e.g., get help when needed, understand changed family dynamics, make meaning of the experience)	**Post- Event-Organizational** (e.g., promote positive reintegration, refer when appropriate, help coworkers/supervisors understand disaster-worker experience)

Returning to Home and Normal Work

- Understand that others are not working at the same pace.

- Be sensitive to family needs, and be aware that family members have had to make changes in your absence.

- Take care in relating your disaster experiences to avoid traumatizing those less familiar with the medical aspects of disasters.

- Keep intolerance for the trivial in check. After working in a disaster, encountering others whose problems and concerns seem trivial can be stressful.

- Resume normal routines as soon as possible.

- Reflect on what you have experienced and learned, and use it to make a positive change in your life.

Roles for the Behavioral Health Professional

Working with and Modeling Leadership

Effective leadership can make or break disaster preparedness, response, and recovery. Behavioral health professionals have numerous important roles with respect to leadership. These include:

- Support and develop positive leadership.

- Formal and informal consultation to leadership on a variety of topics (including personnel issues).

- Dealing with an impaired leader.

- Promote understanding of leadership complexities among line staff.

Additional Roles for Behavioral Health Professionals

Qualified mental health professionals can make significant contributions in disaster settings or the disaster-management field in a variety of ways that include:

- Assuring that the appropriate array of mental health resources are available to victims and their families, responders and their families, and disaster managers at all stages in the event and its aftermath.

- Sensitizing planners and administrators to the psychological aspects of response activities, such as recovery of remains, identification, family notification, and transportation of the injured to distant treatment locations.

- Advising on public-information planning and risk communication—who should say what, to whom, and how.

- Identifying, screening, and training mental health resources.

- Providing crisis counseling, screening, diagnosis, and treatment to those who need these services.

- Developing public-information and educational strategies and materials regarding a wide variety of psychological sequelae.

Roles of and with Others

Behavioral health professionals must be able to work collaboratively with a number of other professionals. A comprehensive and integrated approach will best serve victims and survivors. Other key professionals include school counselors, public health professionals, addiction counselors, pastoral counselors, and chaplains.

In summary, there are many diverse and critical roles that behavioral health professionals can play. At the same time, training, education, organizational role, and temperament make some person/task matches better than others. It is important in all event phases to carefully evaluate where one's contributions can best be made. There is a role for almost everyone, but not everyone is a good match with all roles. It is imperative that all behavioral health professionals interested in the field of disaster management, preparedness, response, and recovery thoughtfully appraise their abilities and temperament to optimize the best functional match. Consulting with colleagues, especially those already in the field, can also be very helpful.

Summary

Everyone who experiences a disaster, whether as a victim or as a responder, is affected by it. However, most of these individuals do **not** develop diagnosable behavioral health disorders.

Early interventions that show the most help are promotion of a sense of safety, promotion of calming, promotion of a sense of self and collective efficacy, promotion of connectedness, and instilling hope. Other interventions, including psychological first aid, are also used. Referrals to behavioral health specialists should be made in cases of severe emotional reactions.

KEY POINTS

 Psychological response to disasters, especially terrorist events, should be anticipated and may outnumber medical consequences.

 Most reactions to disasters are normal responses to severely abnormal situations.

 Disaster responders are not immune from the psychological sequelae of disasters. Their behavior should be monitored for signs of excessive stress.

Threat of Terrorism

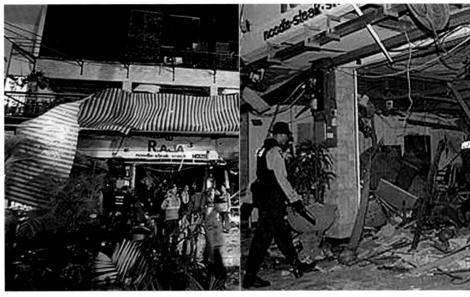

Figs. 26.1, 26.2 Bali Bombing (2002)

CASE SCENARIO

The October 12, 2002, Bali bombings occurred in the tourist district of Kuta on the Indonesian island of Bali. The terrorist attack, carried out by a violent Islamist group, was one of the deadliest terrorist incidents in the history of Indonesia. Approximately 202 individuals were killed, and over 240 people were injured in the attack.

Three bombs were detonated. The first two bombs, a backpack-mounted device carried by a suicide bomber and a large car bomb, were detonated outside popular nightclubs in Kuta. The third bomb was detonated outside the United States consulate in Denpasar with minimal damage.

Introduction

Unique among disaster responses of all types, terrorist and criminal acts add the hazards of intent to harm people, property, the environment, or a combination of these factors. While every disaster medical response is inherently complex and dangerous, only deliberate human action creates an event *designed* to maximize destruction, injury, death, and cultural distress. **With increasing frequency, the perpetrators of these attacks are targeting responders in particular, both in order to hamper efforts to preserve life and to add casualties in a way that touches the targeted culture even more deeply.**

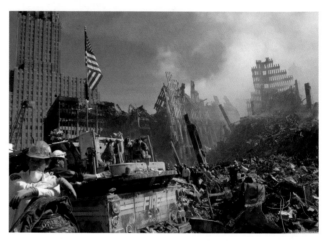

*Fig. 26.3 World Trade Center terrorist attack (2001),
Courtesy of FEMA.*

Terrorist and criminal attacks pose a number of operational and clinical complexities to the medical response. In many cases, the number, nature, and distribution of casualties may be more consistent with combat operations than civilian events. As a result, effective medical operations demand that responders be prepared to adapt both their clinical and operational priorities and activities. This necessity goes far beyond the responder's knowledge of patient care aspects of weapons of mass destruction (explosive, biological, chemical, and radioactive agents).

Terrorism

Terrorism is defined in various ways, but includes the following concepts:

* Criminal use of force or violence indiscriminately targeting a civilian population.

* An effort to coerce an action by a government or group, express an ideology, or carry out revenge.

* The pursuit of a political or cultural objective.

302

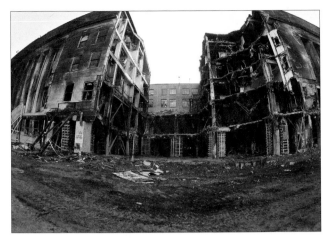

Fig. 26.4 Pentagon terrorist attack (2001),
Courtesy of FEMA.

Terrorist groups may include only a few people with a shared ideology, grievance, or other agenda. In contrast, they may be multi-national groups or networks, as in the case of al Qaeda. Attacks may be state-sponsored, as in the 1988 bombing of Pan Am Flight 103 in the skies over Scotland. Years after the incident, the Libyan government admitted responsibility. A growing number of recent terrorist attacks are the work of single individuals with no direction from, or connection with, any terrorist group.

Examples of terrorist atacks include:

• In 1984, the Rajneesh religious cult used Salmonella bacteria to contaminate local salad bars in Dalles, Oregon. The attack was a trial run for a planned larger attack on the local drinking water supply, intended to help the cult win a number of elected offices. Seven hundred fifty-one (751) individuals were sickened by the agent, purchased from a Seattle, Washington company and cultured in the group's own laboratory.

• In 1995, coordinated chemical attacks were launched in the Tokyo subway system by Aum Shinrikyo, a cult promoting an overthrow of the Japanese government. Although the sarin delivery system performed poorly, 13 individuals died and some 5,000 persons arrived at local hospitals for medical care, many with psychological distress.

• In 2004, coordinated bombings were carried out in Madrid, Spain, in an attempt to influence upcoming national elections. In 13 separate bombings, 191 rail passengers were killed and over 1,700 injured.

• In 2004 in Beslan, Russia, armed separatist militants occupied School Number One for three days and held schoolchildren, teachers, and others hostage, set explosive devices, and held off authorities.

Although precise counts are disputed, it is generally accepted that nearly 1,200 hostages were held, and 396 children and adults were killed. Casualties were a combination of gunshot, blast/shrapnel, and burn injuries. Dehydration and heat-related illnesses complicated the condition of the hostages.

- In 2011, in Oslo, Norway, one individual, a professed right-wing Norwegian citizen with a grievance against his country's immigration policies, carried out a bombing of a government center in Oslo and a mass shooting on an island 40 km (25 miles) away.

Whatever the origins or sentiments of those carrying out terrorist acts, the sophistication and effectiveness of these attacks vary widely. The 2001 attacks on New York's World Trade Center resulted in the collapse of both Towers 1 and 2, damage to many other buildings, and the deaths of over 3,000 individuals. In contrast, the 1993 truck bombing in the underground garage of one of the same towers was meant to topple one building into the other, potentially killing 50,000. Although a van-borne bomb detonated, no collapse occurred. Six individuals were killed and a thousand injured.

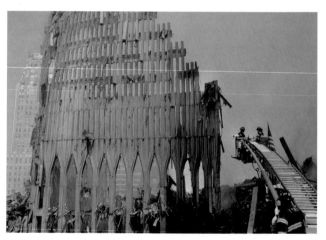

Fig. 26.5 World Trade Center terrorist attack (2001), Courtesy of FEMA.

Criminal Attacks

Not all large-scale attacks are necessarily terrorist acts by accepted definitions. Some are criminal in nature, but don't bear all of the hallmarks of terrorism. For example:

- Colorado's 1999 Columbine High School attack by two students left 15 dead and 24 injured in an incident that involved a combination of shotguns, rifles, handguns, and improvised explosive/incendiary devices. The perpetrators used a small firebomb as a diversion for emergency services, and planted bombs to drive students into their planned field of fire.

- In 2007, a disturbed student staged two sequential shooting attacks at Virginia Tech, killing 32 and wounding another 25 individuals.

Analysis of both school attacks points to perceptions of bullying and ostracism as the motives of the perpetrators. The distinction between terrorism and a large-scale criminal attack deals with motive and the nature of those targeted. The numbers of casualties, the nature of their injuries, and responder actions may be identical. In the interest of simplicity, both are referred to as "terrorism" in this chapter.

Terrorist Devices

Study of worldwide terrorism in recent decades has revealed a number of trends and common features. An understanding of these can help responders operate more safely and effectively. In general, the frequency of use is inversely proportional to the full destructive potential of a mass terror device.

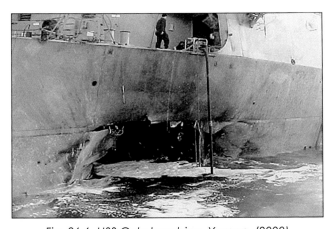

Fig. 26.6 USS Cole bombing, Yemen (2000)

Explosives, firearms, and incendiaries have been the weapons of choice in over 86% of terrorist attacks worldwide during the past four decades. The inclination to use more sophisticated weapons is rare, but never absent. To put it into perspective, 1970-2012 data from the Global Terrorism Database (National Consortium for the Study of Terrorism and Response to Terrorism) includes nearly 106,000 incidents. Chemical, biological, and radioactive incidents combined account for less than a quarter of one percent of attacks. The clear message to the response community: **Don't ignore chemical, biological, and radioactive threats, but understand the comparatively enormous risk of attacks using guns and bombs.**

Terrorists have attempted to obtain or develop biological, chemical, radioactive, and nuclear weapons. At the least likely and most spectacular end of the spectrum would be successful initiation of a nuclear fission weapon. However, the required raw materials, equipment, technical expertise, secrecy, and other considerations probably put this possibility out of the reach of any but a state-sponsored terrorist group. Even the black market procurement of a military nuclear weapon would require considerable sophistication to render it useful to an individual or group.

Terrorist attacks rarely achieve the high numbers of victims hoped for by their planners and perpetrators. However, large attacks have clearly been successfully launched in recent years. It is important to note that a large number of injured, sickened, exposed, and worried-well individuals can easily overwhelm most healthcare systems as was the case in the Tokyo subway attacks.

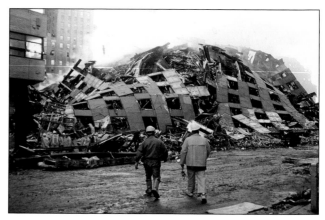

Fig. 26.7 World Trade Center terrorist attack, New York (2001)

The nature of terrorist incidents demands special considerations by all incident managers and responders, including medical personnel.

- The risk of sequential devices and/or attacks should be presumed at every suspected terrorist and criminal attack. The initial event, whether explosive, incendiary, or ambush by gunfire, may be intended to draw in responders and bystanders for a much larger attack.

- Sequential attacks may use the same type of weapon, or may include one or more different types. Attacks may be carried out by the same perpetrator, or may involve multiple gunmen, bombers, or others.

- The incident or scene may be more extensive than other incident types. An explosive, incendiary, chemical, or radioactive attack may immediately impact a very large area. Safe standoff distances may be 2 miles (3 km) or more.

- When buildings, subways, and other facilities are involved, all floors and non-public areas must be considered part of the scene until ruled out. In large buildings or complexes such as those attacked in Oklahoma City and Oslo, Norway, the scene can be much larger than initially appreciated, Extensive resources will be required to search, assess, and secure the area and to locate, treat, and extricate casualties. This can be especially complicated when utility disruption or structural issues preclude use of elevators, building lighting, and other routine services.

RISK ALERT!

Never assume that the elimination of one attacker makes a scene safe from sequential attacks.

A suspected terrorist event demands that scene organization be carefully considered. In a natural disaster or accident, many response operations may be established in the shadow of one or more impacted facilities. The risks of sequential attacks, deliberate spread of contamination, and other factors may make it necessary for medical operations to move much farther away. For example:

- The Incident Command Post and other sites should be established far enough from the scene to avoid undue exposure to risk of a sequential attack.

- Casualty collection, treatment, medical staging, and other areas may have to be a mile or more from the site of the disaster. The need to carry many patients long distances should be considered in incident planning. In many cases, a wheeled device may be used, reducing responder fatigue and allowing patients to be moved by fewer responders.

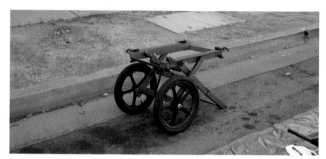

Fig. 26.8 Transport dolly used for backboard.

- Heliports, or landing zones, must be established far enough from the seat of the attack and from ground operations that the helicopter rotor wash will not help distribute chemical, radioactive, or biological agents, disturb crucial evidence, or expose the aircraft unduly to the risk of being targeted by an armed terrorist.

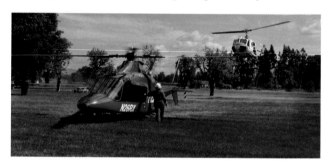

Fig. 26.9 Medical and rescue helicopters are especially vulnerable on approach, landing, and takeoff.

- Security and force protection measures may be in place that seem unduly strict, may be construed to interfere with optimal patient care, or may appear to be insensitive to casualties and bystanders. Responders should understand that these measures may be necessary in order to protect them from sequential attacks or to prevent the escape of perpetrators.

Rescue and medical personnel may need to work closely with tactical law enforcement teams under highly unusual conditions, especially early in a response. This could include extraordinary security checks of responders, limited access to some areas of a scene, and working in close cooperation with specialized tactical teams.

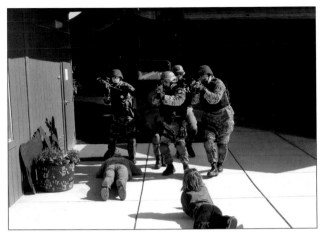

Fig. 26.10 A tactical team may appear to disregard casualties until an area is deemed secure.

Expedient patient transportation may necessitate dragging victims, improvised movements, and other measures that would be considered substandard care in less extreme circumstances. Spinal precautions, splinting, and other measures may need to be delayed in the interest of safety for patients and responders.

- Every responder working a suspected terrorist incident should be well-briefed on the status of the event, all remaining known hazards, safety measures, secure routes in and around the scene, established safe refuge areas, and other operational considerations and medical protocols.

- Patient care practices may be **restricted** because of resource shortages or mass care expediencies, or may be **expanded** to allow some procedures outside of the routine scope of some responders.

- Medical supply demands can be extraordinarily high for these incidents, whether for treatment of large numbers of burns, crush injuries, penetrating trauma, or exposure to chemical or biological agents.

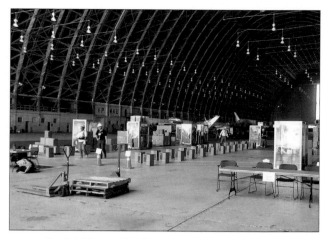

Fig. 26.11 Medical supplies being stockpiled at a staging area.

Personal Protective Equipment (PPE)

Special medical support is essential for responders operating in many types of PPE common to post-attack operations.

- Tactical ballistic equipment may weigh 60 pounds (27 kg) or more and retains body heat, contributing to a high risk of dehydration and heat stress, even in cool atmospheric conditions. The equipment may reduce visibility, mobility, dexterity, and the wearer's ability to judge his/her immediate environment.

- Blast suits are even heavier, and increase all of the hazards described for ballistic equipment. Not all bomb squad teams wear them routinely; however, medical responders should be aware of their hazards.

- Medical providers are accustomed to treating patients in light PPE such as barrier gowns, masks, and eye protection. Higher levels of PPE may be required to safely access, triage, extricate, and possibly treat patients after a terrorist attack. Medical team members should understand the limitations of patient care in this equipment.

- Tactical ballistic equipment can sometimes be adapted to allow for a broad range of patient assessment and care. A stethoscope can be used with many modern tactical helmets, and gloves can often be doffed to facilitate fingertip palpation and performance of procedures requiring a delicate touch.

- Chemical protective suits make it extremely difficult to render medical care to victims. They also subject the wearer to extreme heat stress, slips and falls, and fatigue.

Explosive Devices

Terrorists may employ commercial explosives, military ordnances, homemade formulations, or a combination of any or all of these devices. Explosives may be found in many shapes and consistencies, including solids, liquids, and gels.

Homemade, or improvised, explosives may be manufactured entirely from raw materials, including industrial, agricultural, and household chemicals, beauty supplies, and even human urine. Devices may be camouflaged as an innocent object or hidden in, under, or behind an object or space that belongs in the environment of its placement.

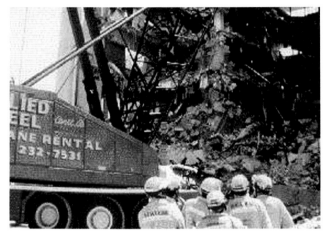

Fig. 26.12 The Murrah Federal Building terrorist bombing, Oklahoma City (1995)

Explosive devices commonly employ more than one material. The truck bomb used in the 1995 Oklahoma City attack included ammonium nitrate fertilizer, commercial nitromethane solvent, diesel fuel, commercial Tovex and ANFO explosives, spools of shock tube, cannon fuse, and blasting caps.

The many variables inherent in the manufacture, preparation, and use of improvised or "homemade" explosives make them highly unpredictable. The devices in the 2010 Times Square "underwear" and "shoe" bombing attempts all failed to detonate as intended because of flawed design or unanticipated conditions.

The types and ranges of injuries encountered after a bombing may vary widely, depending on factors such as:

- **The explosive(s) used.** High explosives such as TNT or ANFO detonate at a rate that creates a primary "blast wave" or "shock wave." This is a highly compressed wall of air, which is disruptive to structures and human tissues. This blast wave can be instantly or nearly-instantly fatal. In contrast, a low explosive such as black powder creates no shock wave, instead creating its injuries by way of its thermal and fragmentation effects.

- **The size of the device:** The larger the device, the greater the injury potential. Responders must remember that a variety of devices may be employed in a single incident, so it is unwise to assume the size or destructive potential of other devices based on those that may have already been detonated or located.

- **The environment:** An open air bomb has a fraction of the destructive power of a similar device planted aboard a bus or train, and an even smaller fraction of one placed in an enclosed structure.

Besides the inherent effects of explosives, responders must be aware of a common terrorist practice of augmenting the antipersonnel properties of their devices by adding such items as:

- Projectiles, such as nails, screws, hardware nuts, and metal debris
- Anticoagulant agents, such as rat poison
- Infectious agents, including using "suicide" bombers infected with hepatitis or other diseases
- Fragments of suicide bombers themselves, such as teeth and bone fragments, which can become high-velocity projectiles.

Explosives are often used in sequence to target emergency responders, investigators, and others who converge on the scene. These may be large or small, disguised as items one might expect to find at the scene, or concealed any place responders might congregate or pass by during their operations. These devices may be detonated by pre-set timers, by using remote command detonation at a time of the bomber's choosing, or by "booby trap." Responders might trigger a booby trap by any of a variety of actions, including:

- Walking or driving through a trip wire across a pressure plate or breaking a light beam
- Transmitting on two-way radio or cell phone
- Opening a door
- Moving an object, including objects normally found at the scene
- Turning a light switch or electrical device on or off

312

BOMB THREAT STAND-OFF CHART

Threat Description Improvised Explosive Device (IED)	Explosives Capacity[1] (TNT Equivalent)	Building Evacuation Distance[2]	Outdoor Evacuation Distance[3]
Pipe Bomb	5 LBS	70 FT/21 M	1200 FT/366 M
Suicide Bomber	20 LBS	110 FT/34 M	1700 FT/518 M
Briefcase/Suitcase	50 LBS	150 FT/46 M	1850 FT/564 M
Car	500 LBS	320 FT/98 M	1900 FT/580 M
SUV/Van	1,000 LBS	400 FT/122 M	2400 FT/732 M
Small Moving Van/ Delivery Truck	4,000 LBS	640 FT/195 M	3800 FT/1159 M
Moving Van/ Water Truck	10,000 LBS	860 FT/263 M	5100 FT/1555 M
Semi-Trailer	60,000 LBS	1570 FT/479 M	9300 FT/2835 M

Bomb Threat Stand-Off Distances (Courtesy of National Counterterrorism Center, 2011)

NOTE: This table is for general emergency planning only. A given building's vulnerability to explosions depends on its construction and composition. The data in these tables may not accurately reflect these variables. Some risk will remain for any persons closer than the Outdoor Evacuation Distance.

[1] Based on maximum volume or weight of explosive (TNT equivalent) that could reasonably fit in a suitcase or vehicle.

[2] Governed by the ability of typical US commercial construction to resist severe damage or collapse following a blast. Performances can vary significantly, however, and buildings should be analyzed by qualified parties when possible.

[3] Governed by the greater of fragment throw distance or glass breakage/falling glass hazard distance. Note that pipe and briefcase bombs assume cased charges that throw fragments farther than vehicle bombs.

Firearms

Firearms are ubiquitous around the world, with a dizzying array of sizes, power, range, magazine capacity, concealability, and other attributes. Assault weapons are popular among terrorists, and are characterized by high rates of fire, large ammunition capacities, and ballistics intended to kill or disable humans. These include fully-automatic weapons that continue firing until the trigger is released or the magazine is empty. Assault weapons are easily obtained in many countries, and may be modified from readily available weapons where assault types are prohibited.

Responders should note that many submachine guns are small enough to be easily concealed on the person of an attacker or in a surprisingly small space at an incident. Even a common semi-automatic handgun can take on characteristics of an assault weapon simply by equipping it with high-capacity magazines, as was the case in the attacks at Columbine High School and the Colorado movie theater.

In skilled hands, a rifle can have an effective range of 1,000 meters or more, a distance that makes it difficult to quickly identify the location of the shooter. Much more commonly, an attacker is less skilled and will rely on high rates and volumes of fire in order to maximize casualties.

Guidelines for tactical medical teams operating in limited ballistic protective equipment include:

- If a weapon or ammunition is discovered, immediately alert law enforcement/security personnel. Avoid moving or handling such items whenever possible.

- When assigned to work in a dark environment, consult with incident command or law enforcement/security regarding any light restriction issues. Excessive or indiscriminate use of flashlights can draw unwanted attention from an assailant. It may be necessary to assess and treat casualties in darkness or dim light.

- If ballistic protective gear is available, consider its use with these cautions:
    - o All ballistic protection has areas of diminished protection and other limitations. Being truly "bullet-proof" is rarely a real possibility.
    - o Ballistic gear is heavy, hot, and fatiguing. It can limit mobility, visibility, and dexterity. Its use is usually best reserved for those trained and practiced in it.

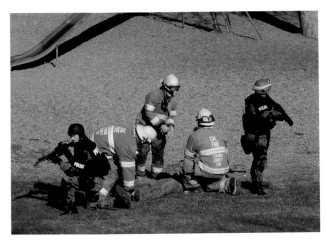

Fig. 26.13 Rescue personnel extricate a casualty under the protection of a tactical law-enforcement team.

When assessing and treating wounded wearing ballistic gear, consider these factors:

- Do not automatically remove body armor in order to visualize or treat injuries. Removal should be based on a balanced decision considering the medical need and the patient's risk of sustaining a subsequent gunshot before he/she can be delivered to a safe location.

- Most body armor is difficult or impossible to cut through with trauma shears. Many vests have a break-away feature to allow quick removal, but cannot be easily replaced on the patient. Other vests have shoulder pads that can be easily removed to allow cutting along the shoulder straps.

- Many high-performance vests have a solid plate over the center chest. This should be considered when assessing mechanism of injury and exposing the patient.

Incendiaries

Incendiaries are the third most common terrorist weapon worldwide. Both explosives and incendiaries are categorized as "energetic materials," and their effects have much in common. Both materials are consumed with significant heat and light, with tremendous potential for damage and injury. **The principal difference is their decomposition rate in a reaction. While explosives typically consume themselves almost instantaneously, incendiaries can sustain the reaction for much longer periods.** Although two comparable materials might release the same amount of energy, the more gradual release of an incendiary makes for a less violent reaction.

While explosives are manufactured and used for their short-duration blast effects, incendiaries are used to ignite, sustain, and, or spread fire. Most incendiaries used by terrorists are gasoline or alcohol-based; however, many other possibilities exist. Homemade thermite, a material that burns briefly and with intense heat, and napalm, which is designed to stick to surfaces as it burns, are well-known incendiaries. Terrorist incendiaries may be constructed, concealed, and initiated just as an explosive might be. These devices tend to be smaller than their explosive counterparts, and may be much more numerous in an attack and at a post-attack scene.

Responder Precautions

- Consider the likelihood of sequential attacks and multiple attackers using similar or different weapons.

- Consult with incident command and/or law enforcement/security personnel for the threat status of all known perpetrators and devices, an assessment of ongoing hazards, safe-zone locations, operating procedures, communications procedures, and other incident-specific details.

- Remain vigilant for evidence of additional devices, including those hidden by or camouflaged as ordinary objects. Immediately notify law enforcement/security of any suspicious object or location.

- Do not move any object, operate any electrical switch, or touch anything unnecessarily.

- Do your utmost to follow established safe routes throughout the scene. If necessary to travel through an unsecured area, place every step deliberately, follow in the footsteps of those who have passed before you, and retrace your steps on the way out. Be alert for any sign of a trip wire, pressure plate, source of a light beam (including invisible infrared), motion sensor, or any other triggering device.

- Consider donning structural firefighting clothing if the risk of additional incendiary devices is deemed high.

- Consider having medical teams accompanied by firefighters with some measure of extinguishment capability.

- When working a post-attack scene, remember that structures may be severely weakened by fire and heat. Floors, walls, supports, and ceilings may be unstable.

Summary

Terrorism follows no rules. The spectrum of potential terrorist threats is limitless. Terrorist and criminal attacks pose significant operational and clinical challenges for medical responders. Terrorists frequently target medical providers responding to the event to increase the morbidity and mortality of the attack.

KEY POINTS

 Explosive devices are the weapons of choice for terrorists.

 The risk of sequential devices and/or attacks should be considered at every suspected terrorist or criminal attack.

 Scene safety is a key priority and often limits the initial medical care at the scene of a terrorist incident.

Disasters and Infectious Diseases

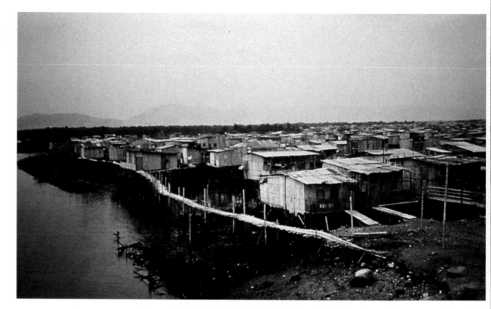

Fig. 27.1 Haiti (2010)

CASE SCENARIO

On October 21, 2010, the Haitian Ministry of Public Health and Population reported a cholera epidemic in the Artibonite Department (region) of Haiti. The epidemic was surprising, as cholera, which is caused by the bacterium *Vibrio cholerae*, had not been reported in Haiti for over a century.

The outbreak followed the powerful earthquake that devastated the country in January 2010. Investigations by public health agencies suggested that contamination upstream of Mirebalais (one of the more severely affected communities) triggered the epidemic.

Introduction

The risk of a significant epidemic is low following most disasters. Infectious deaths following disasters are most commonly caused by measles, diarrheal diseases, and respiratory infections. Any of the following factors may increase the risk of an epidemic:

- Disruption of potable water supply
- Disruption of sanitation (controlled sewage)
- Displacement of populations
- Loss of public health infrastructure or loss of primary medical care infrastructure.

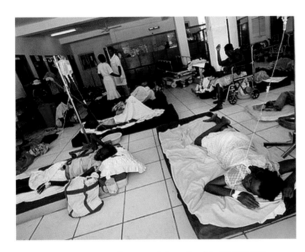

*Fig. 27.2 Cholera epidemic, Haiti (2010),
Courtesy of CDC*

Geopolitical conflicts are more likely to be followed by epidemics than are natural disasters. Much of the elevated risk of epidemics following disasters is related to displacement of populations. In refugee camps, outbreaks of typhoid fever, cholera, and meningitis may occur. Malnutrition, common in many refugee populations, increases the lethality of many infectious diseases, including measles, diarrheal diseases, malaria, and acute respiratory infections (ARI). Contrary to common perceptions, **the risk of dead bodies spreading infectious diseases is very small.**

Pre-disaster Preparedness

Vaccinations

- Medical staff responding to disasters should be current for the following vaccines: tetanus, diphtheria, pertussis, measles, mumps, rubella, hepatitis A and B, influenza, and varicella.

- Responders who work for the developing world should be vaccinated for typhoid fever, which is present in low-income nations around the world.

- Those traveling to tropical Africa or tropical South America should be vaccinated for yellow fever.

- Vaccination for meningococcal meningitis is advised for those traveling to the Sahel of Africa (the belt-like biogeographic zone of transition between the Sahara desert to the north and the Sudanian Savanna to the south), particularly during the dry season (December through June). This vaccine should also be considered for those who will be staying in crowded living situations.

- A single booster of vaccine for polio as an adult, on top of the childhood series, is advised for those traveling to Africa, the Indian subcontinent, and other regions endemic for polio.

- Other vaccinations to consider include rabies, (a viral illness transmitted by bites or scratches of mammals, most commonly dogs) and Japanese encephalitis, a mosquito-borne viral illness present throughout Asia and the Indian subcontinent in rural and farming communities. Since smallpox has been eradicated, smallpox vaccination is not necessary as a routine vaccination unless one is working with researchers who study smallpox or if individuals are exposed to a biowarfare attack with smallpox.

Mosquito Prophylaxis

Mosquitoes and other insects transmit illnesses throughout the tropics. **Approximately half of the world's population is at risk for mosquito-borne illnesses.** Each year, 700 million people become infected with a mosquito-borne illness, most commonly malaria or dengue fever.

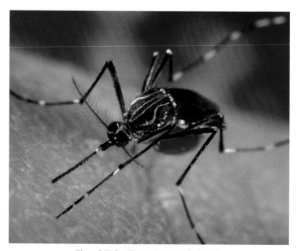

Fig. 27.3 Courtesy of CDC

Those working in regions endemic for malaria should take appropriate prophylaxis:

- Chloroquine or hydroxychloroquine (Plaquenil) in chloroquine-sensitive areas, or
- One of three drugs—atovaquone/proguanil (Malarone), doxycycline, or mefloquine (Larium) in chloroquine-resistant areas.

A listing of all countries in the world with malaria and susceptibility or resistance to chloroquine is listed on the Centers for Disease Control and Prevention (CDC) site.

The use of personal protection measures to reduce insect bites is of paramount importance whether or not one is taking an antimalarial. **There is no vaccine or prophylactic medication available for dengue fever, which is common throughout the tropics in both rural and urban settings.**

The use of personal protection measures markedly reduces risk. DEET (ideally 30-50%) or picaridin 20% should be applied to exposed skin two or three times each day. Permethrin, which has no smell or color, should be applied to all clothes except for underwear at four-week intervals. This will repel insects despite several washes. Wearing long sleeves and long pants offers additional protection. Those in tropical climates should sleep under permethrin-treated mosquito nets.

Post-Response Screening

Diarrhea is common in both residents and visitors in low-income nations. Cautious food selection may partially mitigate risk. Medical responders should avoid tap water, food, or beverages from roadside stands, lettuce and salads, ice, raw meat and seafood, and unpasteurized milk products. Food and drink with lessened risk to cause diarrhea include boiled liquids, bottled water with an intact seal, carbonated beverages, dry foods (e.g., bread), and peeled fruits (e.g., oranges, bananas). Despite following these measures, the risk of diarrhea remains high. All medical staff should have access to an anti-motility agent, such as loperamide, and an antibiotic for self-treatment of diarrhea. A reasonable algorithm is as follows:

Treatment of Diarrhea

- No symptoms – no treatment
- Mild diarrhea – loperamide (Imodium-AD)
- Watery diarrhea – loperamide + antibiotic*
- Fever, blood in stool – medical evaluation (avoid loperamide)

* *For Latin America and Africa: a fluroquinolone, such as ciprofloxacin, 500mg bid. for up to 3 days.*

* *For Southeast Asia and the Indian subcontinent: azithromycin, one gram once or 500mg qd x 2 days in adults.*

Medical responders who have worked in an area of high endemicity for tuberculosis (TB) should get a PPD, a skin test that tests for latent TB (minimum of ten weeks after their return). Alternately, the responder may be tested with an interferon-gamma release test, such as QuantiFERON®-TB Gold. In those testing positive, a nine-month course of isoniazid (INH) markedly reduces the risk of progression from latent to active TB.

Responders with exposure to schistosomiasis (e.g., immersion into a body of fresh water on the continent of Africa) should have a serology drawn for schistosomiasis, also known as bilharzia, a minimum of one month after their most recent exposure. Those testing positive should receive treatment with praziquantel. Additionally, those working for long durations in low-resource settings should consider examination of stool for ova and parasites, even if they are without symptoms.

Specific Infectious Diseases

Measles

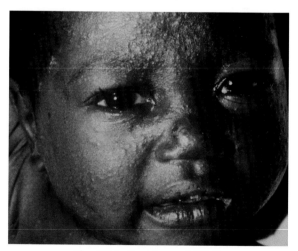

Fig. 27.4 Courtesy of CDC

Measles, a highly-contagious viral illness that is transmitted by respiratory droplets, is common in displaced populations in the developing world. **Symptoms include fever and "the three C's": cough, *coryza* (runny nose), and conjunctivitis.** A characteristic maculopapular erythematous rash, usually evident 3-5 days after the first signs of illness, begins on the head and spreads downward. The case-fatality rate (CFR) in stable populations is about 2%; however, in refugee populations, the CFR often exceeds 5%.

Measles can cause acute *kwashiorkor* (protein-deficient malnutrition) in children with borderline malnourishment and can worsen vitamin A deficiency, potentially leading to *xerophthalmia* (extreme dryness and thickening of the conjunctiva), blindness, and premature death. When possible, efforts to vaccinate those affected by a disaster should be coordinated with the local Expanded Program for Immunizations (EPI), a World Health Organization (WHO) program usually administered by a nation's Ministry of Health.

In the acute emergency phase, immunization for measles is the top vaccine priority, particularly for children in regions with low rates of immunization. Additionally, vitamin A should be given to children over nine months of age, which decreases mortality by 30-50%.

Diarrheal Diseases

As many as 25-50% of deaths in refugee settings are due to diarrheal diseases. In children under five years of age, persistent diarrhea (over 14 days in duration) is associated with living with other young children and malnutrition. Rather than persistent infection with a single organism, many children with persistent diarrhea are infected with multiple organisms, either simultaneously or sequentially. Bacteria causing chronic diarrhea in refugee settings include *Campylobacter* species, enterotoxigenic *Escherichia coli*, and *Shigella*. Protozoan organisms include *Cryptosporidium*.

Cholera is characterized by high-volume watery diarrhea. Although non-cholera causes of diarrhea are probably responsible for more deaths than cholera, cholera can lead to abrupt and catastrophic epidemics with high CFRs. During the Rwandan genocide in 1994, between 500,000 and 800,000 Rwandan Hutus crossed into the Democratic Republic of Congo (DRC) in a one-week period. Approximately 50,000 refugees died in a one-month period from infectious diseases. A significant percentage of the high mortality was due to an epidemic of cholera.

According to a May 2011 report from the United Nations, the epidemic of cholera in Haiti that followed the January 2010 earthquake resulted in 581,000 cases and 7,400 deaths, with a CFR of 2.4%. Risk factors for cholera include:

- Polluted water sources

- Absence of controlled sewage facilities

- Shared water containers and cooking pots

- Lack of soap

The primary treatment of cholera is hydration. This can usually be accomplished orally. IV rehydration may be necessary in patients who are vomiting or comatose.

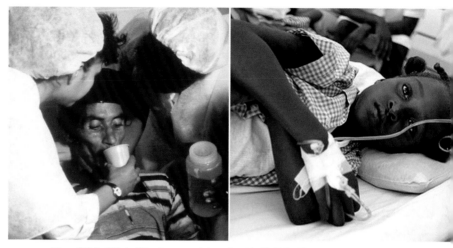

Figs. 27.5, 27.6 Cholera epidemic, Haiti (2010), Courtesy of CDC

Cholera Treatment

Antibiotic regimens include:

- Azithromycin 1 gram once.
- Doxycycline 300 mg in a single dose.
- Tetracycline 500 mg qid x 3 days.
- Children: azithromycin 20mg/kg in single dose
- Alternatives include ampicillin and erythromycin.

Antibiotic treatment of cholera is not mandatory, but a short (1-3 day) course of antibiotics will lessen the volume of diarrhea in severe cholera. Additionally, antibiotics will shorten the duration during which V. *cholerae 01* is excreted in the stool. A course of antibiotics usually causes a cessation of diarrhea within 48 hours and has been shown to result in a shortened hospitalization.

A secure source of potable water and controlled sewage reduces the risk of diseases transmitted by the fecal-oral route, including cholera. Additional preventative measures include the provision of hand washing facilities, reducing overcrowding, and supplemental feeding.

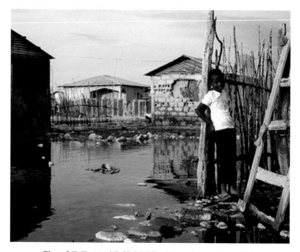

Fig. 27.7 Haiti (2010), Courtesy of CDC

Acute Respiratory Infections

Among refugee populations, acute respiratory infections (ARI) are one of the three most common causes of death. ARI may be divided into upper (AURI) and lower (ALRI) infections. AURI affect the nose, sinuses, middle ear, larynx, or pharynx. ALRI affect the trachea, bronchi, or lungs. The great majority of severe illnesses and deaths due to ARI are caused by ALRI, most commonly pneumonia. Almost all severe episodes of ALRI occur in children, the elderly, or the immunosuppressed.

Between one-quarter and one-half of cases of pneumonia in children are viral in etiology, the most common viral pathogens being human respiratory syncytial virus (RSV), influenza, and parainfluenza. At least half of causes of pneumonia in children are bacterial, some of which are secondary infections of viral infections, including measles, influenza, and RSV. Bacterial pneumonia is associated with increased severity and higher CFRs relative to viral infections. Given that distinction between bacterial and viral pneumonia is often difficult to make in a post-disaster or refugee setting, antibiotic treatment is often indicated even in the absence of pathogen identification.

Malaria

Malaria is the infection with a protozoan organism, *Plasmodium*. **Typical symptoms include fever, chills, and diaphoresis.** Five species of *Plasmodium* commonly cause human infection. *Plasmodium falciparum* is the most common and the most severe. The vector for malaria is the *Anopheles* mosquito. **Measures that reduce exposure to mosquitoes will reduce the incidence of malaria.**

The incidence of malaria has been found to increase dramatically following some disasters. For example, malaria was markedly more common following the 1991 earthquake in Limón, Costa Rica. This is postulated to have been caused by changes in human behavior (e.g., sleeping outdoors), cessation of ordinary malaria control measures, and changes in habitat favorable to mosquito breeding (increased standing water).

Civil unrest has led to increases in the incidence of malaria in a number of countries, including Burundi and Afghanistan. Displaced populations who live in makeshift housing are more likely to be bitten by mosquitoes. The severity of their malaria infections is compounded by malnutrition and concomitant illnesses. Refugees and displaced populations suffer elevated morbidity and mortality from malaria when they originate from regions with no or low incidence of malaria and transit into regions of high-endemicity.

Personal protective measures against malaria include:

- Insect repellent (30-50% DEET)
- Long sleeves/long pants
- Use of an insecticide-treated bed net
- Apply permethrin to clothing

325

The availability of rapid point-of-care diagnostic tests, (e.g., BinaxNOW®), offers an alternative to traditional thick and thin smear microscopy. In large epidemics, it is logistically impossible to confirm each suspected case of malaria by either a rapid diagnostic test (RDT) or microscopy. After an RDT survey establishes that malaria is the cause of an epidemic and a clinical case definition has been established, mass treatment of those meeting the clinical case definition should be instigated. Pregnant women and children under the age of five years should receive top priority as they are at elevated risk of severe illness and death. Note: most RDT remain positive for about one-to-two weeks after completion of therapy.

Those who test positive for malaria or meet the clinical case definition should receive prompt treatment with an appropriate anti-malarial regimen.

- In chloroquine-sensitive regions, chloroquine remains an effective anti-malarial drug.

- **In regions in which malaria is resistant to chloroquine and in areas with unknown resistance, individuals diagnosed with malaria should receive artemisinin-based combination therapy (ACT).**
  Options include:

   o Artemether-lumefantrine
   o Artesunate plus amodiaquine
   o Artesunate plus mefloquine
   o Artesunate plus sulfadoxine-pyrimethamine
   o Dihydroartemisinin plus piperaquine.

- **Utilizing permethrin-treated bed nets markedly reduces risk of malaria.**

- Eliminating standing pools of water will reduce available breeding sites for mosquitoes and hence reduce the incidence of malaria.

Typhoid Fever

Typhoid fever, caused by the bacterium *Salmonella typhi*, is transmitted by the fecal-oral route. Following an incubation period of 1-2 weeks, symptoms can be protean. Classic symptoms include:

- Fever

- Malaise

- Diffuse abdominal pain

- Constipation

TREATMENT ALERT!

Malaria treatment depends on whether the case occurs in a chloroquine-sensitive region or a chloroquine-resistant region.

Findings on physical exam include:

- Fever

- Abdominal tenderness

- Bradycardia

- In 30% of cases, a faint, salmon-colored, blanching, maculopapular rash, known as *rose spots,* which can be difficult to detect in dark-skinned people.

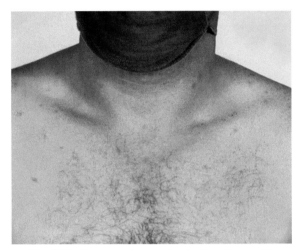

Fig. 27.8 Rose spots on chest of patient with typhoid fever, Courtesy of CDC

The most accurate method of diagnosis is culture of bone marrow aspirate, which is 90% sensitive, but this is not usually practical in a post-disaster or refugee setting. Diagnosis can also be made by culture of multiple blood samples, intestinal secretions (vomitus or duodenal aspirate), or stool. Stool cultures alone yield a sensitivity of less than 50%. The once-popular Widal test, which measures agglutinating antibodies against H and O antigens of *S. typhi,* is neither sensitive nor specific and should not be utilized.

Antibiotic treatment reduces CFR from 20-30% to approximately 1%. Options include ciprofloxacin, levofloxacin, ceftriaxone, or azithromycin. Chloramphenicol is still used in some low-resource settings. Surgery is indicated in cases of intestinal perforation.

Meningitis

Outbreaks of meningococcal meningitis occur in populations, including refugees, in or near Africa's semiarid Sahel, also known as the *meningitis belt.* Outbreaks are more common during the dry season, which begins in December and ends in June. The incidence of 15 or more cases per 100,000 population per week in two successive weeks has a high predictive value for an epidemic.

Usual symptoms are:

- Fever
- Severe headache
- Photophobia
- Nausea
- Vomiting
- Stiff neck
- A purpuric rash may be present.

Treatment options include cefotaxime, ceftriaxone, penicillin G, ampicillin, moxifloxacin, and chloramphenicol. In the event of a laboratory-confirmed case of meningococcal meningitis, a mass vaccination program should be initiated, with the highest priority being the family and close community contacts of identified cases.

Leptospirosis

Typhoons, heavy rains, and floods elevate the risk of leptospirosis, also known as rat fever. The disease is caused by a spirochete that is excreted in the urine of rats, other rodents, and other animals. Symptoms include jaundice and fever. A single dose of doxycycline, 200 mg (or weekly doses in the event of a prolonged exposure), may prevent infection with leptospirosis, but clinical trials regarding efficacy have had conflicting results.

Coccidioidomycosis

Coccidioidomycosis is a fungal disease caused by *Coccidioides immitis*, which is native to the San Joaquin Valley of California, USA, or *C. posadasii*, which is found in the southwestern US, northern Mexico, and some locations in South and Central America. The fungus lives in soil. Infection is usually transmitted by inhalation of airborne spores. The most common presentation is a self-limited respiratory tract infection.

Case Study

Following the 1994 Northridge, California earthquake, an outbreak of 203 cases of coccidioidomycosis, including three fatalities, was identified. The organism was in all likelihood transmitted by dust clouds raised by the landslides caused by the earthquake.

The peak of disease onset occurred two weeks after the earthquake. Case-study control data identified age over 40 years and exposure to a dust cloud as risk factors for developing acute coccidioidomycosis.

Tetanus

Tetanus remains common in the developing world, causing an estimated 300,000 to 500,000 deaths annually. Tetanus has been noted in affected populations following disasters in regions in which routine vaccination is infrequent or absent. Risk is particularly elevated following disasters such as earthquakes and floods. Tetanus, caused by the bacterium *Clostridium tetani*, may occur after wounds are contaminated with dirt, feces, or saliva. **The absence of a wound does not exclude the diagnosis of tetanus. No wound is found in as many as 20% of tetanus cases.** Tetanus is not transmitted person-to-person.

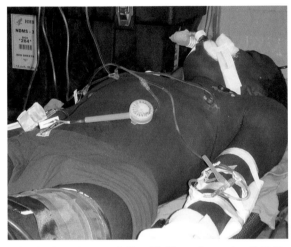

Fig. 27.9 Tetanus victim, Haiti earthquake (2010)

No laboratory data provide a definitive diagnosis of tetanus. Diagnosis is based on clinical findings. **The WHO definition of tetanus includes trismus (lockjaw) or risus sardonicus (a fixed leering grin) or painful muscle contractions in a patient with a history of a potentially contaminated wound, such as a puncture wound, burn, crush injury, gangrene, or other traumatic injury.** Four clinical types of tetanus are recognized: generalized, localized, cephalic, and neonatal.

Tetanus vaccine should be administered immediately to those with traumatic injuries unless they have received a booster of tetanus toxoid within the previous ten years. Ideally, tetanus immune globulin (TIG), in addition to tetanus toxoid, is administered to those individuals with injuries who have not been vaccinated for tetanus. However, following a wide-scale disaster, medical teams may not have a sufficient supply of TIG to administer it to all injured patients without a history of immunization for tetanus.

Care for those with generalized tetanus consists of:

- Passive immunization with TIG
- Active immunization with tetanus toxoid
- An antibiotic such as metronidazole
- Wound irrigation and debridement
- Heavy sedation
- Ventilatory support.
- Magnesium infusion has been found to control the need for other drugs to reduce muscle spasm and cardiovascular instability.

Endemic Infectious Diseases

Although an acute increase in tuberculosis (TB) is not seen following disasters, TB is endemic throughout the developing world. Spread may be facilitated by crowded living conditions. Patients with active tuberculosis often present for care following disasters, although their illness is not related to the disaster. Those with suspected active pulmonary TB (e.g., a patient with cough for over three weeks, fever, and weight loss) should be isolated. Ideally, those with active TB should be referred to a facility able to provide long-term care. Routine treatment for active pulmonary TB consists of four anti-TB medications for two months, followed by two anti-TB medications for four months.

Exposure of Medical Staff to Infectious Diseases

Sleep deprivation and urgency may result in an elevated rate of needle stick injuries among medical staff. **HIV post-exposure prophylaxis (PEP) medications should accompany medical teams operating in an area with a significant prevalence of HIV.**

In the event of caring for a patient with meningococcal meningitis, staff with close contact for at least four hours, or who have performed invasive procedures such as endotracheal intubation or suctioning, should receive prophylaxis with an appropriate antibiotic. The most convenient medication for adults is ciprofloxacin 500 mg once if not ciprofloxacin-resistant. Other options include ceftriaxone 250 mg IM, rifampin 600 mg every 12 hours X 4 doses for four days, or spiramycin 500 mg every six hours for five days.

Summary

Infectious diseases are common in disasters, although the risk of an epidemic is low if adequate water supplies and sanitation facilities exist in the areas affected by the disaster.

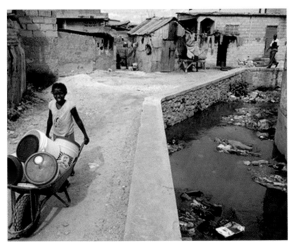

Fig. 27.10 Haiti earthquake (2010),
Courtesy of CDC

Immunization of medical providers responding to disasters is critical for responder safety, particularly in low-income countries lacking adequate pre-disaster medical care.

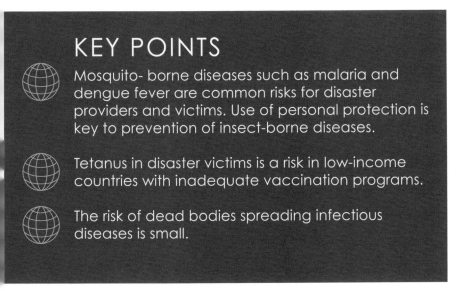

KEY POINTS

Mosquito- borne diseases such as malaria and dengue fever are common risks for disaster providers and victims. Use of personal protection is key to prevention of insect-borne diseases.

Tetanus in disaster victims is a risk in low-income countries with inadequate vaccination programs.

The risk of dead bodies spreading infectious diseases is small.

Anesthesia
in Austere Environments

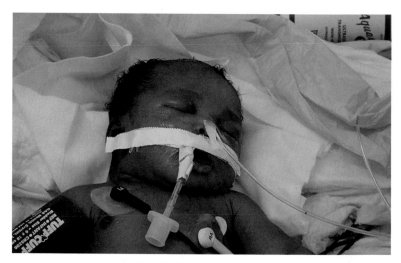

Fig. 28.1 Haiti earthquake (2010)

CASE SCENARIO

Urgent airway interventions are common in all disasters, but particularly in disasters such as earthquakes where victims are trapped under collapsed buildings and sustain significant crush injuries to the face and thorax. During the Haiti earthquake in 2010, many victims required emergency intubation, both for traumatic and non-traumatic conditions. Intubation and anesthesia for urgent life-saving procedures present unique challenges for medical providers in austere environments. Children are a particular challenge.

Introduction

An austere environment may have limited resources, personnel, and equipment, causing greater challenges in the provision of anesthetic care. Uncommon climate and environmental conditions generally force medical personnel to practice outside their normal range. This chapter offers basic and practical information as groundwork for the successful administration of anesthesia in any disaster situation.

Pre-anesthetic Considerations

History and Physical Examination

In disaster situations, an abbreviated history and physical are often necessary as medical providers must treat life-threatening injuries rapidly.

Volume Assessment

Preoperative fluid status should be assessed in all patients. Anesthetizing a severely hypovolemic patient can cause intractable, potentially fatal, hypotension. An intravenous fluid bolus may be necessary prior to intravenous (IV) sedation.

Pre-anesthetic medication

- Intravenous histamine (H$_2$) antagonist, (e.g., cimetidine or ranitidine)
  All patients for emergency surgery are considered to have full stomachs and are at increased risk for gastric aspiration.

- IV opioids for pain control

- Benzodiazepines for severe anxiety

- Anticholinergics (e.g., atropine, glycopyrrolate) to prevent parasympathetically-mediated phenomena such as bradycardia and hypersecretion.

AMPLE History:

- Allergies
- Medications
- Past medical history
- Last meal
- Environment/ Event

Abbreviated Physical Examination:

- Measure and record vital signs
- Perform thorough airway evaluation
- Examine heart and lungs
- Evaluate for hemorrhage and hypovolemia
- Assess for chest, abdominal, and other injuries

ABCs of Resuscitation

- Airway maintenance with cervical-spine protection

- Breathing and ventilation

- Circulation with control of hemorrhage

- Disability or neurological status

- Exposure (undress the patient) and Environment (maintain patient's temperature)

Airway Management

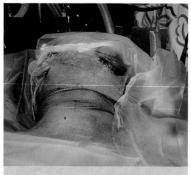

Fig. 28.2 *Blunt injury to the neck with airway swelling*

- Airway patency must be assured using techniques such as neck extension, jaw thrust, chin lift, and oral or nasal airway devices.

- A laryngeal mask airway (LMA) may be used to support an open airway, but aspiration is possible. An appropriately sized LMA may be inserted into the hypopharynx after anesthetic induction. The LMA forms a loose-fitting seal around the glottic opening, allowing positive pressure and spontaneous ventilation.

- Orotracheal intubation provides a definitive airway, with a cuffed endotracheal tube (ETT) precluding aspiration.

- Intubation is indicated in specific surgeries, or when a difficult mask fit, prolonged controlled ventilation, or prone surgery is encountered.

- The sniffing position (head elevated on blankets) and generous mouth opening facilitates a view of the larynx. Laryngoscope (left hand) should displace the tongue to the left. The tongue and pharyngeal soft tissues should be lifted (not levered) to afford a view of the larynx.

- A 7.0 mm or 8.0 mm internal diameter ETT is generally employed in adults.

- Pediatric endotracheal tubes are generally sized by the following formula: (age / 4) + 3.

- **The diameter of the child's pinky gives a good estimate of the appropriate size ETT.**

- External pressure over the cricoid cartilage may provide better visualization of the glottis and prevent aspiration (Sellick maneuver).

- It may be necessary to use a stylet in the ETT to achieve better mechanical advantage.

- The ETT pilot balloon should be inflated until there is no air leak from the trachea when a positive pressure breath of less than 30 cm H_2O pressure is applied.

- In children, cuffless ETTs or low inflation pressures (i.e. tolerance of air leak at less than 24 cm H_2O pressure) are preferred.

- End tidal CO_2 monitoring and auscultation of equal breath sounds over both lung fields will verify correct placement of the ETT.

- Other techniques exist for placement of an ETT, including awake intubation, nasal intubation, and tracheostomy. If the tracheal intubation is expected to be difficult, awake intubation should be considered.

Classes of Anesthesia

In general, the most practical and valuable anesthetic techniques in "field" medicine (austere setting) include ketamine, conscious sedation, regional anesthesia, and occasionally general anesthesia. **Ketamine is one of the most frequently used agents in environments without electricity, supplemental oxygen, and highly trained personnel.** One can carry out a moderately safe and reliable anesthetic and perform a large variety of operations solely with the use of ketamine (without the need for endotracheal intubation or assisted ventilation).

> **TREATMENT ALERT!**
>
> **Field Debridement:**
>
> **Ketamine 1.0-1.5 mg/kg IM or IV**

Ketamine

Ketamine is a short-acting, potentially hallucinogenic anesthetic.

Advantages

- Rare need for intubation or assisted ventilation
- Can be given either intramuscularly (IM), or intravenously (IV) via bolus or infusion
- Stable compound—no refrigeration necessary
- Bronchodilatation
- Rapid recovery
- Titratable

Disadvantages

- May be associated with laryngospasm
- Risk of dissociative experiences and dysphoria
- Increased secretions, bronchospasm
- Raises intracranial pressure, not suitable in patients with head trauma or known intracranial pathology (i.e., tumor, bleeding)

Half-Life

- 10-15 minutes
- Elimination half-life: 2 to 3 hours
- Clinical effect lasts 10 to 30 minutes, depending on dose.

DOSING AND ADMINISTRATION (ADULTS)

1. Sedation and Analgesia:

- 0.2 to 0.75 mg/kg initially
- 5 to 20 mcg/kg/min maintenance

2. Induction and Maintenance:

- IV induction doses of 1-2 mg/kg
- Maintenance doses of 0.1–0.5 mg/minute or one half of the full induction dose, repeated as needed. Continuous maintenance infusion of 10-30 mcg/kg/min is also employed.

Ketamine*

Ketamine, a non-barbiturate anesthetic/analgesic agent, is used for induction and maintenance of general anesthesia, sedation, and analgesia (pain relief). It is a rapid-acting general anesthetic producing an anesthetic state characterized by profound analgesia, normal or slightly enhanced skeletal muscle tone, cardiovascular and respiratory stimulation, and occasionally, a transient and minimal respiratory depression. The anesthetic state produced by ketamine has been termed "dissociative anesthesia" in that it appears to selectively interrupt association pathways of the brain before producing somatesthetic sensory blockade.

EMERGENCE REACTIONS

Some patients describe the effects of ketamine as a pleasant, dream-like state, vivid imagery, hallucinations, and emergence delirium. Others explain the effects as unpleasant, with confusion, excitement, and irrational behavior. A sensation of body detachment or "floating in space" is also described. Dreaming and flashbacks can sometimes persist for many days.

Emergence reactions are experienced by approximately 12% of patients. Elderly patients and pediatric patients under the age of 15 are least likely to experience emergence reactions. Patients with a history of abnormal dreaming and personality disorders are more likely to experience emergence reactions.

Conscious Sedation

Conscious sedation is a minimally depressed level of consciousness that retains the patient's ability to maintain a patent airway and consciously respond appropriately to physical stimulation and verbal commands.

Drugs Used for Conscious Sedation (Adults)

- Meperidine (Demerol) 50-150 mg

- Morphine 5-15 mg

- Fentanyl (Sublimaze) 0.025-0.15 mg

- Diazepam (Valium) 5-20 mg

- Midazolam (Versed) 1-5 mg

- Droperidol (Inapsine) 0.5-5.0 mg

Advantages
- No intubation needed
- Rapid reversal
- Ability to converse with patient
- Rapid recovery

Disadvantages
- Narrow therapeutic window
- Patient may require emergency intubation

NOTE: Propofol is **not** included in the list of drugs used for conscious sedation. Propofol is best administered by experienced anesthesia personnel as this agent provides moderate to deep sedation, and continuous airway monitoring and support are necessary.

Drugs Used to Reverse Conscious Sedation

- Opiate reversal: naloxone (Narcan) 0.4-2.0 mg; may repeat in 20 minutes

- Benzodiazepine reversal: flumazenil (Romazicon) 1 mg (short duration of action)

Regional Anesthesia

Regional anesthetic (RA) techniques include major neuraxial blockade (spinal, epidural, and caudal), plexus blocks (cervical, brachial, and lumbosacral), individual nerve blocks, and local infiltration.

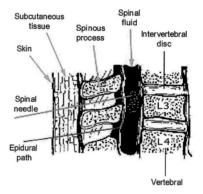

Fig.28.3 Regional anesthetic techniques

Advantages

- Most orthopedic and extremity surgery can be performed safely with RA.

- Epidural and caudal anesthesia can be established with a continuous catheter or single-dose technique.

- Spinal anesthesia is administered as a single dose of local anesthesia directly into the cerebrospinal fluid, whereas epidural anesthesia entails the administration of a local anesthetic solution in the epidural space, posterior to the ligamentum flavum.

- Regional anesthesia is generally contraindicated in patients with major coagulation abnormalities or who are on anticoagulation therapy.

Disadvantages

- Disadvantages of RA include:
    - Local anesthetic toxicity
    - Incomplete neural blockade, obliging intraoperative change to general anesthesia
    - Vasodilatation (autonomic blockade)
    - Hypotension
    - Bradycardia

- High thoracic neural blockade (T2, T3, and T4) will paralyze thoracoabdominal and intercostal muscles. This high anesthetic level impairs deep breathing and effective coughing and will diminish respiratory function.

- Regional anesthesia techniques may take more time to administer than general anesthesia and may not be suitable when time is essential.

338

Brachial Plexus Anesthesia

- Complete anesthesia of the shoulder, arm, or hand may be provided by administration of local anesthesia around the brachial plexus.

- Ultrasound-guided administration of local anesthesia around the supraclavicular brachial plexus provides complete anesthesia of the shoulder, upper arm, elbow, lower arm, and hand. With ultrasound guidance, risk of pneumothorax or subclavian arterial puncture is low.

- Axillary block via transarterial or ultrasound technique provides safe, effective anesthesia to the elbow, forearm, and hand.

Fig. 28.4 Portable ultrasound

Lumbosacral Plexus and Individual Lower Extremity Blocks

- Ultrasound-guided femoral nerve block provides rapid anesthesia or analgesia to the anterior leg, knee, and saphenous distribution of the lower leg/foot.

- Saphenous nerve block alone provides effective lower leg analgesia without loss of quadriceps muscle strength.

- Sciatic nerve block at the subgluteal level provides posterior leg, knee, and foot anesthesia. At the popliteal fossa, muscle strength of the hamstring is spared while still providing effective analgesia to the lower leg and foot.

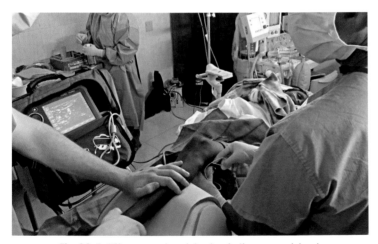

Fig.28.5 Ultrasound-guided sciatic nerve block

Ankle block is a readily-placed volume block of the superficial and deep peroneal, sural, saphenous, and tibial nerves. Epinephrine is avoided as a local anesthetic adjuvant for ankle block.

General Anesthesia

General anesthesia (GA) implies a lack of consciousness and loss of protective airway reflexes. Although it holds several advantages over other anesthetic techniques, GA may not be practical in some field situations.

Advantages

- When endotracheal intubation is used, it secures and protects the airway and assures adequate ventilation.
- Muscle relaxation is practical in patients who are under GA.
- Rapid induction of GA is accomplished with IV or inhalation induction, and the level and interval of anesthesia can be easily controlled.

Disadvantages

- Loss of airway reflexes
- Risk of gastric aspiration
- Hypotension (especially with induction and deeper levels of anesthesia)
- Tachycardia (during endotracheal intubation/extubation and emergence from anesthesia)
- Hypertension (during airway instrumentation after induction and withdrawal of GA)
- Most head, neck, chest, and upper abdominal surgery will require GA.

Management of General Anesthesia

Induction

Rapid-sequence induction or "awake" intubation is generally required for all patients at high risk for gastric aspiration. The following clinical scenarios are associated with increased aspiration risk:

- Trauma
- Bowel obstruction
- Ileus
- Symptomatic hiatal hernia
- Severe gastro-esophageal reflux
- Second or third trimester of pregnancy
- Morbid obesity

Three basic induction techniques are used: IV, inhalation, and IM induction. Inhalation anesthesia is usually not available in the field, and IM anesthesia is less reliable.

Intravenous induction is accomplished with injection of a potent short-acting hypnotic agent administered intravenously over 10 – 15 seconds in a bolus, such as:

- Ketamine (~1.5 mg/kg)
- Propofol (~ 0.5—2 mg/kg)
- Thiopental (~ 4 mg/kg)
- Etomidate (~ 0.3 mg/kg)

The patient may or may not continue to breathe after injection. Usually, the anesthetist should determine that establishment of artificial respiration with a bag-valve mask is possible. If endotracheal intubation is planned, a muscle relaxant may then be administered. In the setting of an emergency operation, a rapid sequence induction (RSI) is performed, in which the induction agent (etomidate) is immediately followed by administration of a fast-acting muscle relaxant (succinylcholine). Attempts at ventilation are avoided and cricoid pressure is held until the ETT tube is accurately positioned, thus avoiding gastric insufflation and risk of aspiration. Vital signs should be monitored frequently—at least every five minutes for the duration of the anesthetic.

Field Anesthesia Equipment

- Laryngoscope
- Bag-valve mask
- Suction equipment
- Nasal/oral airways
- Endotracheal tubes
- Cricothyroidotomy sets
- Syringes/needles
- McGill forceps
- Drugs: local anesthetics, ketamine
- Stethoscope
- Blood pressure cuff
- Pulse oximeter

Complications of General Anesthesia

- Hypotension (need to rule out other etiologies of hypotension, including blood loss, sepsis, and spinal cord injury)
- Hypoxemia
  - o Airway obstruction
  - o Laryngospasm/bronchospasm
  - o Gastric aspiration
- Atelectasis
- Hypothermia
  - o Cold IV fluids
  - o Vasodilatation
  - o Evaporation

Failed attempts at intubation

- If the use of direct laryngoscopy has failed to intubate the trachea, attempts at ventilation or placement of an LMA may keep the patient sufficiently oxygenated until definitive surgical airway management is performed.

- Needle cricothyroidotomy involves placement of a 12 g or 14 g cannula though the cricothyroid membrane. Although oxygenation is possible through a needle cricothyroidotomy, ventilation is difficult and hypercapnia is common.

- If a patient cannot be intubated safely and requires a definitive airway for ventilation, a surgical cricothyroidotomy may be performed by experienced medical providers. A horizontal or vertical incision may be utilized. Elective tracheostomy should be performed as soon as possible.

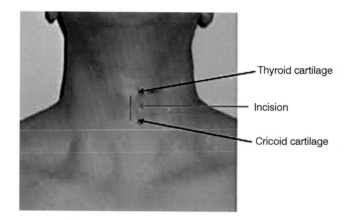

Fig. 28.6

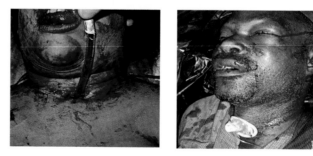

Figs. 28.7, 28.8 An endotracheal tube (left image) or tracheostomy tube (right image) may be used for emergency surgical cricothyroidotomy.

Summary

Austere environments with limited resources present special challenges in the provision of anesthetic care for disaster victims. The most practical and valuable anesthetic techniques in austere environments include ketamine, conscious sedation, regional anesthesia, and less frequently general anesthesia.

KEY POINTS

 Signs of a difficult airway may alter choice of anesthetic agents.

 Ketamine is one of the most frequently-used agents in austere environments.

 Many orthopedic and extremity surgeries can be performed under regional anesthesia.

Care of the Dead, Their Families, and the Responders

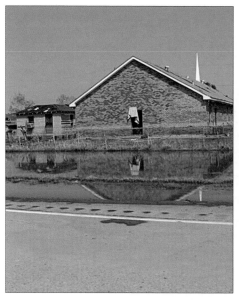

*Fig. 29.1 Flooding from Hurricane Katrina,
New Orleans (2005)*

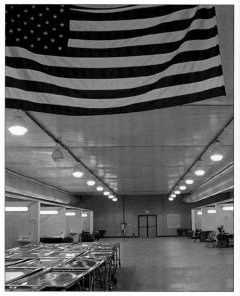

*Fig. 29.2 Temporary Morgue,
Carville, Louisiana (2005)*

CASE SCENARIO

On August 29, 2005, Hurricane Katrina struck New Orleans, Louisiana. Initial hurricane damage was further complicated by failures of the levees and flood walls protecting New Orleans and its suburbs, resulting in devastating flooding of the city. Disaster Mortuary Response Teams (DMORT) were deployed to New Orleans as the New Orleans morgue was destroyed. A temporary morgue was established by DMORT in St. Gabriel, Louisiana and later moved to a newly-constructed facility in Carville, Louisiana. DMORT closed operations at this temporary morgue on March 1, 2006.

Introduction

Disasters of any type take a heavy toll on all those involved. Mass fatalities, such as those caused by terrorist acts, present unique circumstances that change the way one deals with deceased victims. Depending on the nature and scope of the disaster and its location, specialized DMORT teams may be available to handle the remains of victims. However, responders must have an understanding of the principles that guide this work.

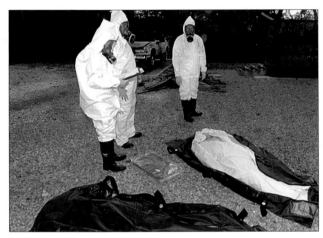

Fig. 29.3 Training simulating mass-fatality disaster

A Disaster Mortuary Response Team (DMORT) generally includes 25 primary responders. Teams include funeral directors, law enforcement agents, fingerprint experts, photographers, pathologists, medical examiners, radiologists, mental health staff, and support personnel. In the US, there are 10 teams, one for each FEMA (Federal Emergency Management Agency) region. There are also additional teams, including one that specializes in decontamination of human remains known as DMORT WMD (Weapons of Mass Destruction).

- The first priority is the safety of the responders.

- Scene security is of utmost importance to keep out unauthorized personnel and prevent the removal and/or relocation of potential evidence prior to documentation.

- The entire scene must be completely documented with charts, diagrams, and photographs before removal of the bodies from the scene. Responders should keep deceased individuals' personal belongings with the remains (on the bodies) to assist in their identification.

- Because the site of a terrorist attack is a crime scene, responders must maintain the <u>chain-of-custody</u> of evidence when dealing with personal effects and other materials found with and around victims.

- Responders should realize that the handling of deceased victims of a disaster presents psychological, emotional, and even legal complications for recovery personnel. Not only must they face the personal trauma of recovering human remains, but they also have obligations to the deceased's next of kin.

- Responder teams should acknowledge and honor cultural and religious beliefs, burial customs, traditions, and legal restrictions of the community they are serving.

Safety of Responders

The safety of responders is the first priority in any recovery situation.

- Secure the safety of the immediate environment using on-site disaster response personnel, including engineers when necessary, before attempting to retrieve bodies.

- In disasters caused by explosions, multiple sharp objects may be present in the clothing or embedded in the victims. Responders must take extra care to prevent injuries to themselves and further trauma to bodies as they prepare them for transport.

- Non-hazardous objects found near the body, including glasses, clothing, airplane parts, etc., should be properly documented with diagrams and photographs prior to removal. Chain-of-custody must be strictly followed. All must be bagged, tagged, and secured for documentation and preservation.

- Handle casualties contaminated with chemical and/or biological agents with appropriate precautions. Physical protection such as personal protective equipment (PPE) is the most effective prophylaxis against chemical and biological agents.

- In case a victim should be found alive, do not take contaminated victims into any medical facility without decontaminating them first. Whenever possible, this should be done by specially trained staff. **The removal of shoes and clothing reduces most hazards up to 95%.** All clothing removed must be triple-bagged in red biohazard bags.

Construction of a Temporary Morgue

When it is not feasible or possible to transport dead bodies to a morgue, responders should set up a temporary field morgue.

- Bodies should be refrigerated as soon as possible at 2°-4° C (35° – 40° F). Refrigerated trailers, known as reefers, can be used for this purpose. Approximately 20 bodies can be put into a 53-foot refrigerated semi-trailer.

- Until bodies can be refrigerated, they should be kept in a cool area and placed upon sealed concrete or metal surfaces – never on wood.

- Out of respect for possible religious and cultural customs, plus maintaining evidence, no embalming preservatives should be used.

- When refrigeration is not available and based on the number of dead, mass burial may be necessary to prevent disease as a last resort.

Care of Bodies

- Once responders have retrieved bodies from the casualty scene, the remains should be placed into heavy-duty body bags and removed to a temporary morgue.

- Bodies believed to be contaminated with toxic agents should be brought to a decontamination station located away from any occupied areas. At this point, the toxin(s) should be determined and a decontamination procedure initiated by trained hazardous-material specialists.

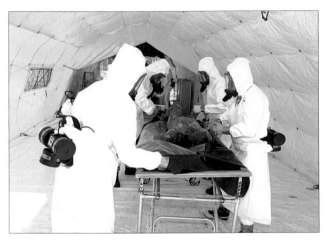

Fig. 29.4 Training simulating mass-fatality disaster

- Until responders are able to make positive identification of individual victims, they should tag each body using a consistent identification system.

- Responders should try to keep fragmented body parts referenced to each other as much as possible. Fragmented parts should never be bagged with a body with the assumption they go together.

RISK ALERT!

As part of the response to the Oklahoma City, Oklahoma bombing in 1998, a local produce company donated refrigerated trucks for the temporary storage of bodies. In spite of its generosity, the company went out of business shortly afterwards. The public felt uncomfortable buying produce from trucks that had been used to store dead bodies.

To avoid this, companies providing trucks for this purpose must have the company name and logo covered with tarps or other materials that will block out the identification of the company.

Preservation of Personal Effects

Chain-of-custody knows where each article and body is at all times, with proper documentation by date, time, and initials of each person who has had possession of that article or body.

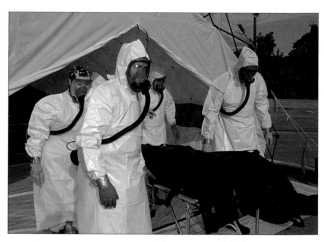

Fig. 29.5 Training simulating mass-fatality disaster

It is critical to preserve the personal effects of deceased individuals and to tag them with the same identifier used for the victim so that they can be identified later. Personal effects may range from wallets and photographs to credit cards, jewelry, laptop computers, and cash. Items like these are helpful in identifying victims and must be stored safely so that they can eventually be returned to family members.

- Each article of clothing should be placed in a separate plastic bag, double or triple bagged as necessary, and tagged with the same identifier as the victim.

- For longer-term storage, wet articles should be air-dried and placed into paper bags so they will not mildew.

- Personnel should avoid cross-contamination of human remains and personal effects by putting one item only in each bag.

In a terrorist attack, bodies, clothing, and personal effects are considered potential evidence. <u>Chain-of-custody</u> must be maintained for each body and personal item to ensure admission in court during the legal process.

Identification of Individual Bodies

"Positive identification" is the identification of an individual ruling out all possibilities of a mistake. There are four methods commonly used to make positive identifications:

- Fingerprints

- Dental records

- Medical implants, such as pacemakers

- DNA (Vendors must all use the same format so that all information can be cross-referenced to the same database.)

Personnel must exercise caution in relying solely on visual identification by next of kin. Many misidentifications have been made because family members have not looked at the deceased closely, or because injuries may have caused swelling or facial trauma that make it difficult to accurately identify the individual. Visual identifications must be supported by other means as well.

Items such as wallets, jewelry, distinctive tattoos, clothing, and other personal effects may point to a particular victim, but must never be used to make a positive identification.

Cultural and Familial Considerations

When dealing with the dead, responders should give primary consideration to the deceased individual's and family's religious beliefs and cultural customs whenever possible. Cultural sensitivity in dealing with the dead and their families is critical to the success of any recovery mission.

For example, in Jewish culture, it is traditional for the burial to take place as soon as possible, even on the same day of the death, but no more than two nights after the death. In traditional Chinese culture, improper funeral arrangements are felt to inflict ill fortune and disaster upon the family of the deceased. Responders, such as members of DMORT, will take time to talk to and work with family members of the deceased to honor local customs whenever possible.

A major task of responders is to support the family, to facilitate the process of making a positive identification of the victim, and, through this, to help families move forward in the grieving process.

All responders must be debriefed after the event or prior to their returning home. Failure to debrief responders before they demobilize and return home can cause them to suffer emotional trauma months or even years in the future.

Summary

Care of the dead and their families present unique challenges for medical providers. DMORT teams are a valuable component of disaster medical response. DMORT teams are composed of multi-disciplinary experts to meet all the requirements for identification and care of dead victims, regardless of the complexity of disasters.

KEY POINTS

 The safety of responders is the key priority in any recovery situation.

 Chain-of-custody must be maintained for each body and personal items in all disasters involving fatalities.

 Cultural sensitivity in dealing with the dead and their families is critical to the success of any disaster response.

Ultrasound in Disasters

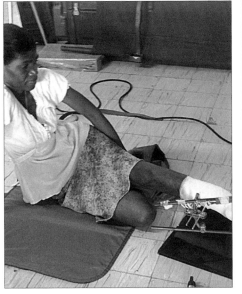 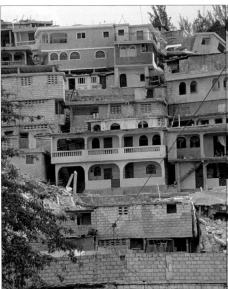

Figs. 30.1, 30.2 Field hospital, Haiti earthquake (2010)

CASE SCENARIO

The Haiti earthquake of 2010 devastated most of the medical infrastructure in Port-au-Prince, including all major hospitals and clinics. Diagnostic imaging equipment was severely limited prior to the earthquake in many medical facilities due to cost and personnel constraints. International field hospitals and mobile medical units responding to the disaster region utilized portable ultrasounds extensively in the care of victims.

Introduction

In mass casualty situations, regardless of existing resources, affected areas quickly become "resource poor" settings due to the number of victims. It is important to fully utilize low-cost diagnostic tools and implement time- saving measures in disasters. Effective use of diagnostic imaging modalities, such as ultrasound, will facilitate triage and emergency care in a timely fashion and will optimize the ability of any given system to respond to disaster needs.

Ultrasound technology continues to improve, making it easily portable, user friendly, and ubiquitous in emergency settings. Thus, ultrasound is becoming an indispensable tool for disaster medical responders. In this setting, ultrasound use can be thought of as "life-saving" as well as "time-saving." These advantages were found to be indispensible in caring for the victims of the earthquake in Haiti.

Ultrasound: A "life-saving" intervention

Airway

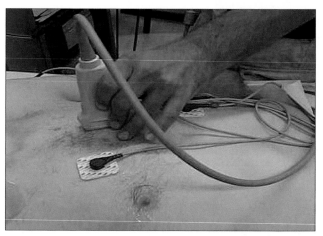

Fig. 30.3 Proper probe position to assess lung sliding in the supine patient.

In mass casualty settings, establishing a secure airway is often required. Confirmation with traditional methods such as chest x-ray or end-tidal CO_2 may be logistically challenging, and these tools are often un- available. Lung ultrasound can be used to assess the presence of lung sliding. Bilateral lung sliding indicates a correctly placed tube. Similarly, the absence of sliding on the left might indicate a right mainstem intubation, or no sliding an esophageal intubation. Further- more, the linear probe can be used to guide intubation by visual- izing the passage of the tube through the trachea. When placed just superior to the cricothyroid membrane, the shimmering reflection of the tube within the tracheal space (and not lateral distending the esophagus) can be very helpful. However, occasionally the esophagus can be directly posterior to the trachea and confirming placement with lung sliding is essential.

To do this, use the linear (5-10 MHz) transducer placed perpendicularly to the ribs to view the 3rd-4th intercostal space. Breaths will cause the hyperechoic pleural line to slide or shimmer with inspiration/expiration, indicating the pleural surfaces are opposed and the lung is being well-ventilated.

Breathing

Even in the non-intubated patient, a pneumothorax can be ruled out with the same maneuver. By placing the probe in the same position as above, the shimmering of the pleural line demonstrates that under the footprint of the probe the two pleural surfaces are touching. When the two lines of pleura are touching, you will see comet tails. These are caused by the sound reverberating between the two opposed lines of pleura. They should shimmer under the probe and radiate down a few centimeters. They should not extend all the way to the end of the probe field. The more rib spaces that are interrogated, the more sensitive lung ultrasound is for ruling out a pneumothorax. Obviously, in a patient who is hypotensive and in respiratory distress, it is not necessary to interrogate the entire chest. A large tension pneumothorax should be fairly obvious with only evaluation of the most superior lung segments (anterior in a supine patient and superior in an upright patient). The absence of lung sliding indicates a pneumothorax, although there are a few conditions that can cause false-positives (adhesions, scar, right-mainstem intubation), so clinical correlation in the absence of lung sliding is essential.

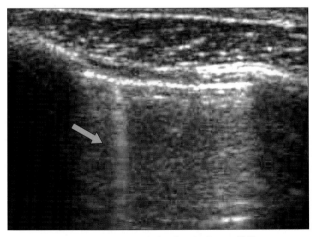

Fig. 30.4 Comet tails indicate lung sliding

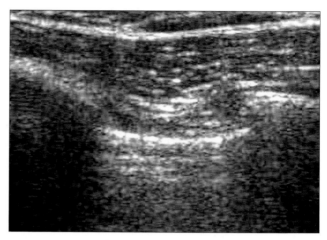

Fig. 30.5 No comet tails

The curvilinear probe can also be used in the mid-posterior axillary line over the inferior chest to identify fluid in the pleural cavity causing respiratory compromise.

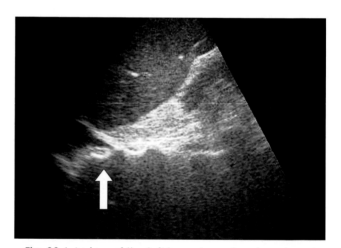

Fig. 30.6 A view of the left lower lung showing pleural effusion. The extension of the spine visible in the far field behind the lung, known as the "spine sign" (white arrow), indicates fluid in the pleural space. If no fluid is present, this area of lung will mirror the soft tissue under the diaphragm.

Circulation

A cardiac ultrasound can demonstrate the presence or absence of cardiac activity. Additionally, pericardial effusions causing tamponade physiology can be identified.

To perform cardiac ultrasound, place the curvilinear probe in the 4th intercostal space and point the probe marker toward the left hip. An effusion will appear anechoic and surround the heart. Care should be taken that the fluid crosses anteriorly to the descending thoracic aorta (Image 5). A large left sided pleural effusion can be mistaken for a pericardial effusion. A pleural effusion (Image 6) should taper to and not cross the descending aorta (white arrow).

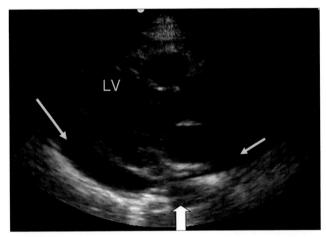

Fig. 30.7 Pericardial effusion (yellow arrows) cross in front of descending aorta.

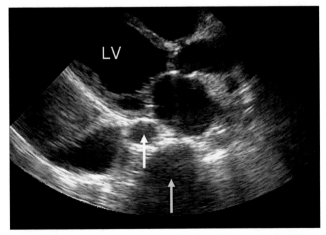

Fig. 30.8 Large left pleural effusion does not cross the descending aorta.

Finally, when evaluating circulation, the Focused Assessment with Sonography for Trauma (FAST) exam will indicate free fluid in the peritoneal cavity as an explanation of hypotension. The FAST exam includes 4 views: the right upper quadrant (Morrison's pouch), left upper quadrant, pelvic (pouch of Douglas) and cardiac views. Free fluid in one of these areas, in the appropriate setting, would indicate the possible need for surgical intervention.

The Fast Exam

The fast exam is performed as follows:

Right upper quadrant (RUQ)

Place the curvilinear probe in the midaxillary line between the 7th-9th rib spaces. Adjust caudal or cephalad to bring the interface between the liver and kidney into view. Free fluid will appear as an anechoic stripe between the two structures. This view is negative if you image the entire kidney (both poles) and the interface between the liver and kidney and diaphragm and do not see free fluid.

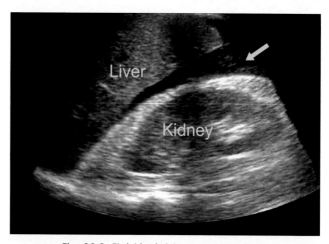

Fig. 30.9 Fluid in right upper quadrant

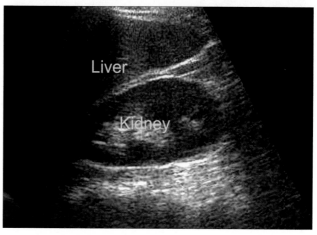

Fig. 30.10 Normal right upper quadrant

Left upper quadrant (LUQ)

Similar to the previous view, place the probe in the midaxillary line between the 7th-9th ribs and adjust as necessary. You are looking for fluid at either pole of the kidney, between the kidney and spleen, or under the diaphragm. The spleen is more superior and more posterior than the liver, so your probe will have to be farther back and higher up on the patient's flank.

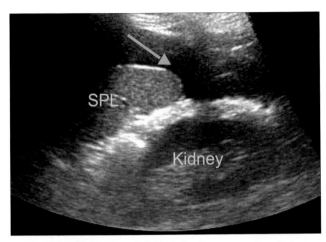

Fig. 30.11 Free fluid in left upper quadrant

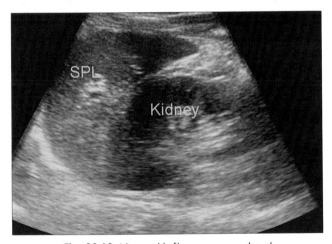

Fig. 30.12 Normal left upper quadrant

357

Pelvic

Using the curvilinear probe, place it in a transverse orientation just superior to the pubic symphysis. Without moving the probe, rock your hand back and forth until you have imaged from the most inferior to the most superior view of the bladder. You are looking for anechoic fluid posterior to the bladder. Then rotate the probe 90 degrees to look in a sagittal direction. Similarly, rock your hand back and forth to view the entire bladder, and look posterior to the bladder for free fluid.

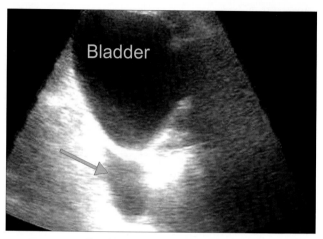

Fig. 30.13 Free fluid in pelvis

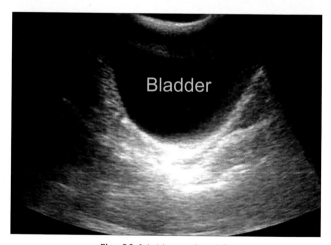

Fig. 30.14 Normal pelvis

Cardiac view

While the cardiac views (parasternal long and parasternal short) are sufficient to assess for a pericardial effusion, using the subxiphoid view can often be quicker. With the same probe used for the three other views, place the probe over the epigastric or RUQ area and shoot toward the patient's left shoulder. Be sure to increase your depth. Press down slightly on the probe to bring the heart into view. Look for fluid around the four chambers.

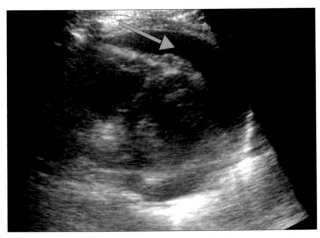

Fig. 30.15 Pericardial effusion

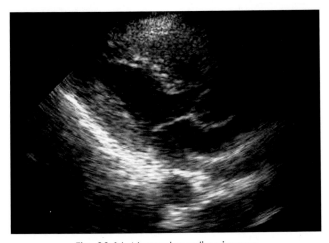

Fig. 30.16 Normal cardiac image

Ultrasound: A "time- saving" intervention

During a mass casualty event, it can be difficult to accurately predict the severity of individuals' injuries or the resources needed to treat them. Ultrasound can assist in these situations. The use of ultrasound to assess the optic-nerve diameter is a good example. Clinically, it might not be possible to distinguish between those with head injuries who would benefit from neurosurgical intervention and those without clinically significant intracranial pathology. Using the ultrasound to measure the optic-nerve diameter has been shown to accurately predict intracranial pressure. A diameter > 5 mm, measured 3 mm from the globe, correlates to increased intracranial pressure seen on computed tomography (CT).

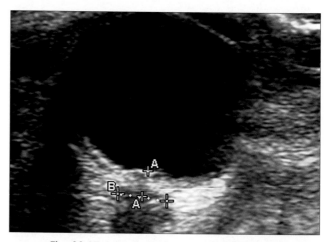

Fig. 30.17 Increased intracranial presssure

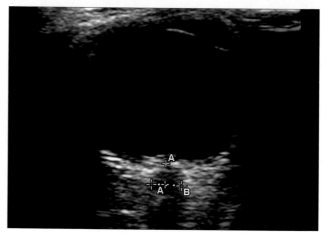

Fig. 30.18 Normal intracranial pressure

Similarly, pregnant women who suffer injuries need either urgent obstetric interventions or close monitoring. Using the curvilinear probe to evaluate the fetal heart rate can help to quickly treat patients when time is of the essence.

To calculate the fetal heart rate, first identify the cardiac activity of the fetus (Image 17). Then use M-mode over the beating heart. Measure the time between two consecutive peaks or troughs. This is the fetal heart rate (Image 18).

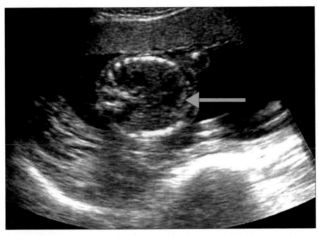

Fig. 30.19 Thorax of fetus with heart (yellow arrow)

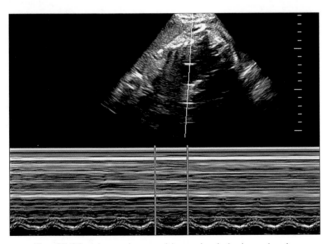

Fig. 30.20 M-mode used to calculate heart rate

Many patients in disasters present with musculoskeletal complaints. The demand for x-rays and limited resources would likely mean these patients would have long waits and take up vital resources. However, using the linear probe along areas of deformity would allow for quick diagnosis and treatment. Likewise, one can distinguish between lacerations and open fractures quickly.

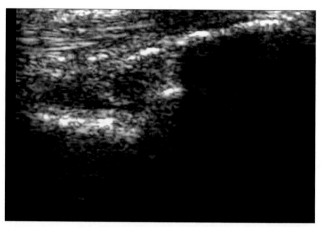

Fig. 30.21 Long bone fracture

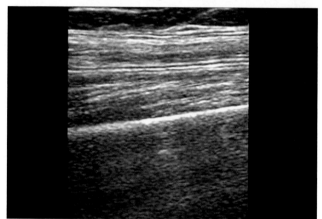

Fig. 30.22 Normal long bone

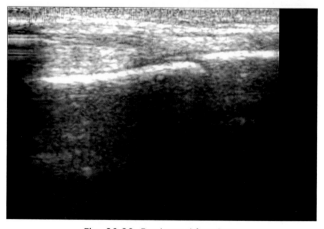

Fig. 30.23 Reduced fracture

Summary

Disaster events are unique situations in which rapid triage and resource utilization become paramount. The use of ultrasound in triage, diagnosis, and treatment greatly benefits both providers and patients. Basic ultrasound skills for life-saving interventions should be routinely taught to disaster response teams. As comfort and skill increases, staff should be trained on time-saving uses.

KEY POINTS

 Portable ultrasound is a valuable asset in the care of disaster victims, particularly in mobile medical facilities.

 Multiple specialties can utilize portable ultrasound in the care of patients seen in disaster settings (obstetrics, orthopedics, critical care).

 All disaster medical providers should learn the basics of ultrasound use.